A REAL FOOD ALPHABET

SANDRINE PEREZ OF NOURISHING OUR CHILDREN

APPRECIATION

Mohammad Naser offered invaluable layout design advice. Kathy Kramer of The Weston A. Price Foundation provided critical proofreading support! Dennis Sookikian and Steve McInally of UBuildABook helped with every step of the printing workflow. The following sponsors generously donated toward the creation of this book:

Terrie and Ray Atkin	
Biodynamic Wellness	biodynamicwellness.com
Carolyn Erickson	realfoodcarolyn.com
Green Pasture Products	greenpastureproducts.com
Homemade Mommy	homemademommy.net
Sally Fallon Morell of New Trends Publishing	newtrends.com
Perfect Supplements	perfectsupplements.com
Radiant Life	radiantlifecatalog.com
Drs. John and Catherine Rott, DNM, D.PSc	yldist.com/royallyredeemed
The Weston A. Price Foundation	westonaprice.org

CREDIT

Sandrine Perez wrote the text and captured a number of photographs that appear in this book, as well as purchased stock photography. Cynthia Castro C. Henriquez photographed her son Elliot for the anchovies page. Please note that no part of this book may be reproduced or transmitted in any form or by any means without prior written consent from Sandrine Perez. Printed by UBuildABook in the United States of America.
ISBN-13: 978-0-578-40238-3.

DEDICATION

For Max, my beloved nephew, and his parents Paul and Emma whose courage has touched me deeply.

Aa Almonds

We soak nuts and seeds in unrefined salt overnight so they're easier to digest.

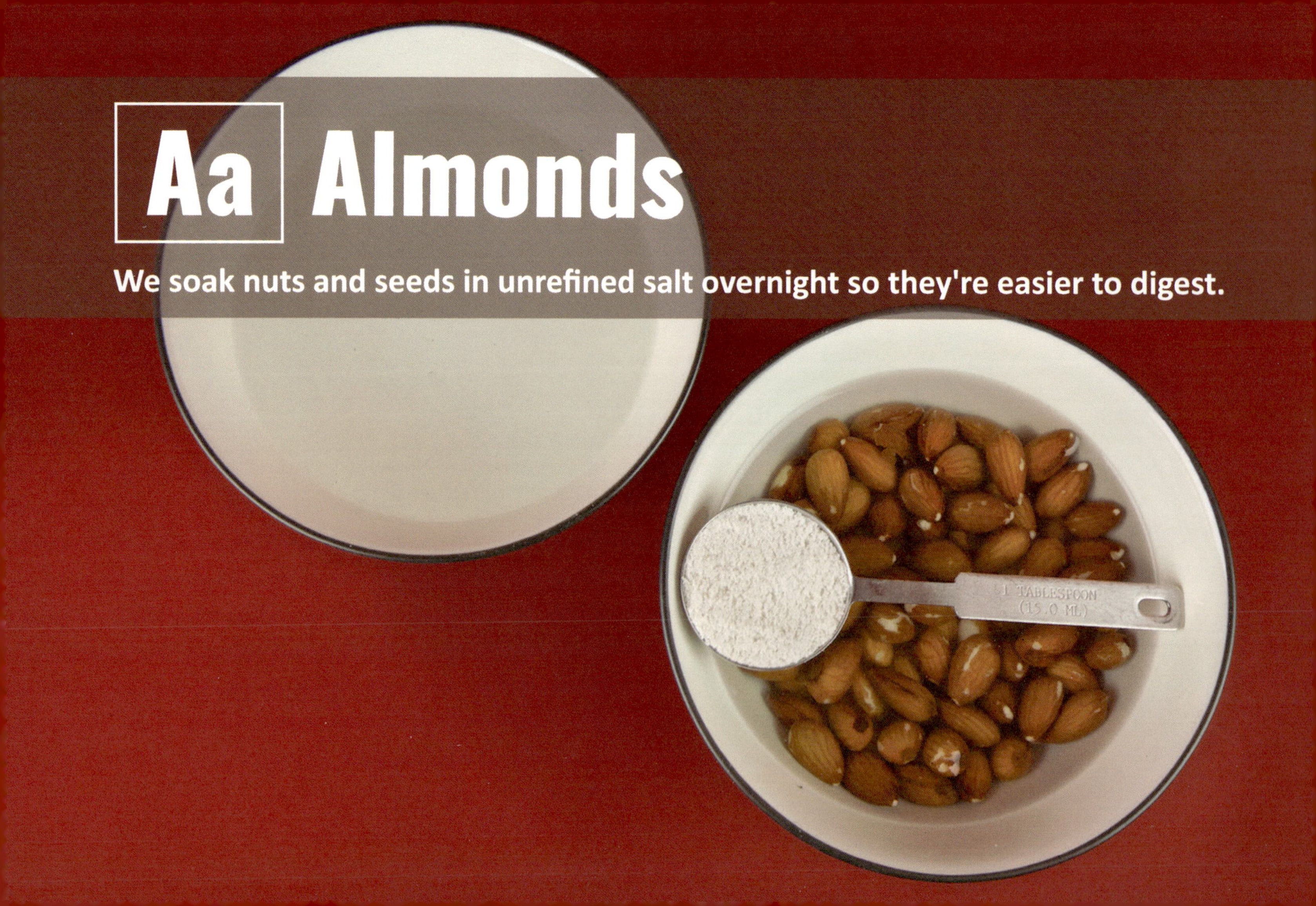

Aa Anchovies

Anchovies are rich in healthy fats, vitamins and minerals. Elliot ate the whole bag!

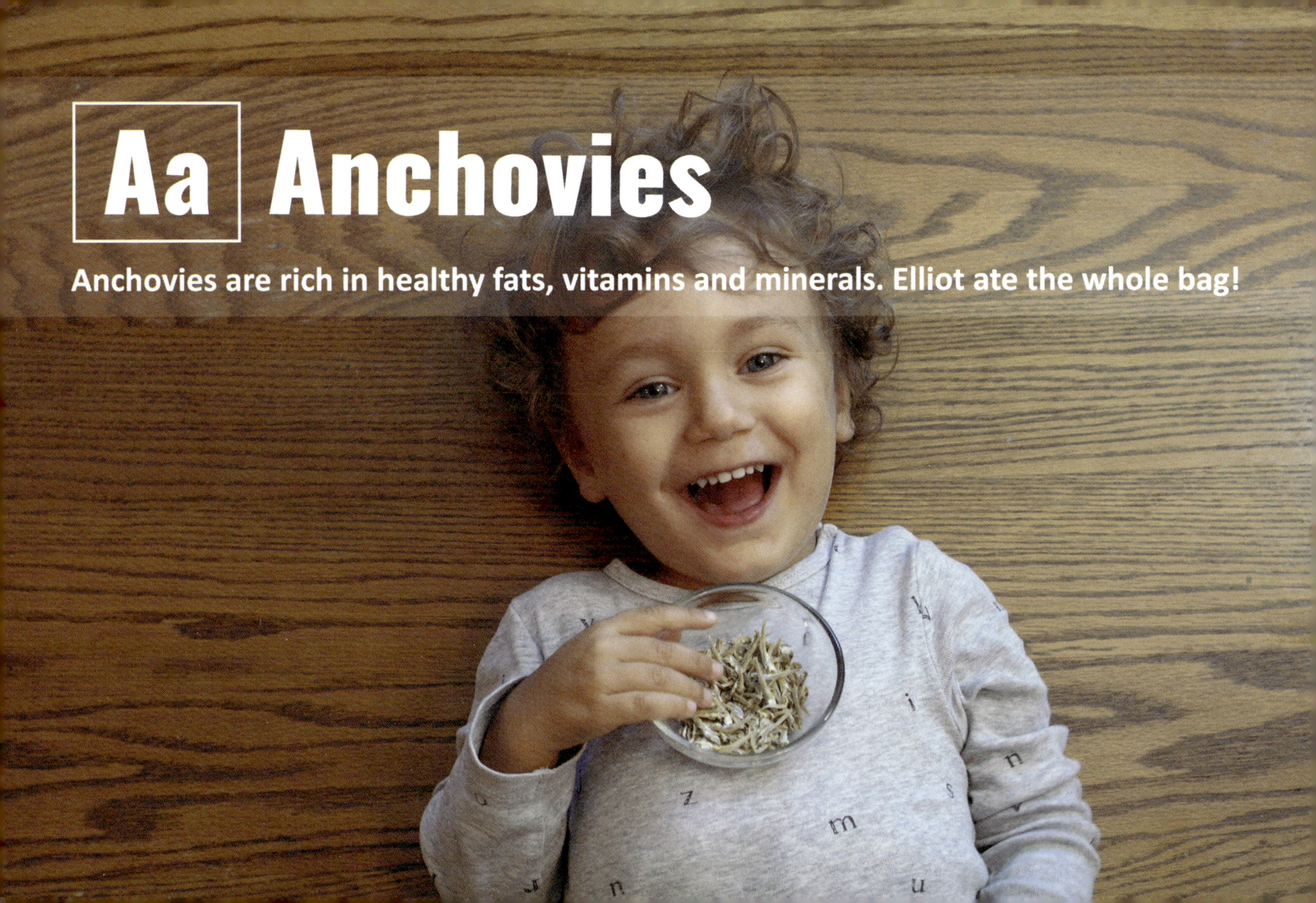

Bb Bone Broth

Broth made with bones from pasture-raised and wild-caught animals.

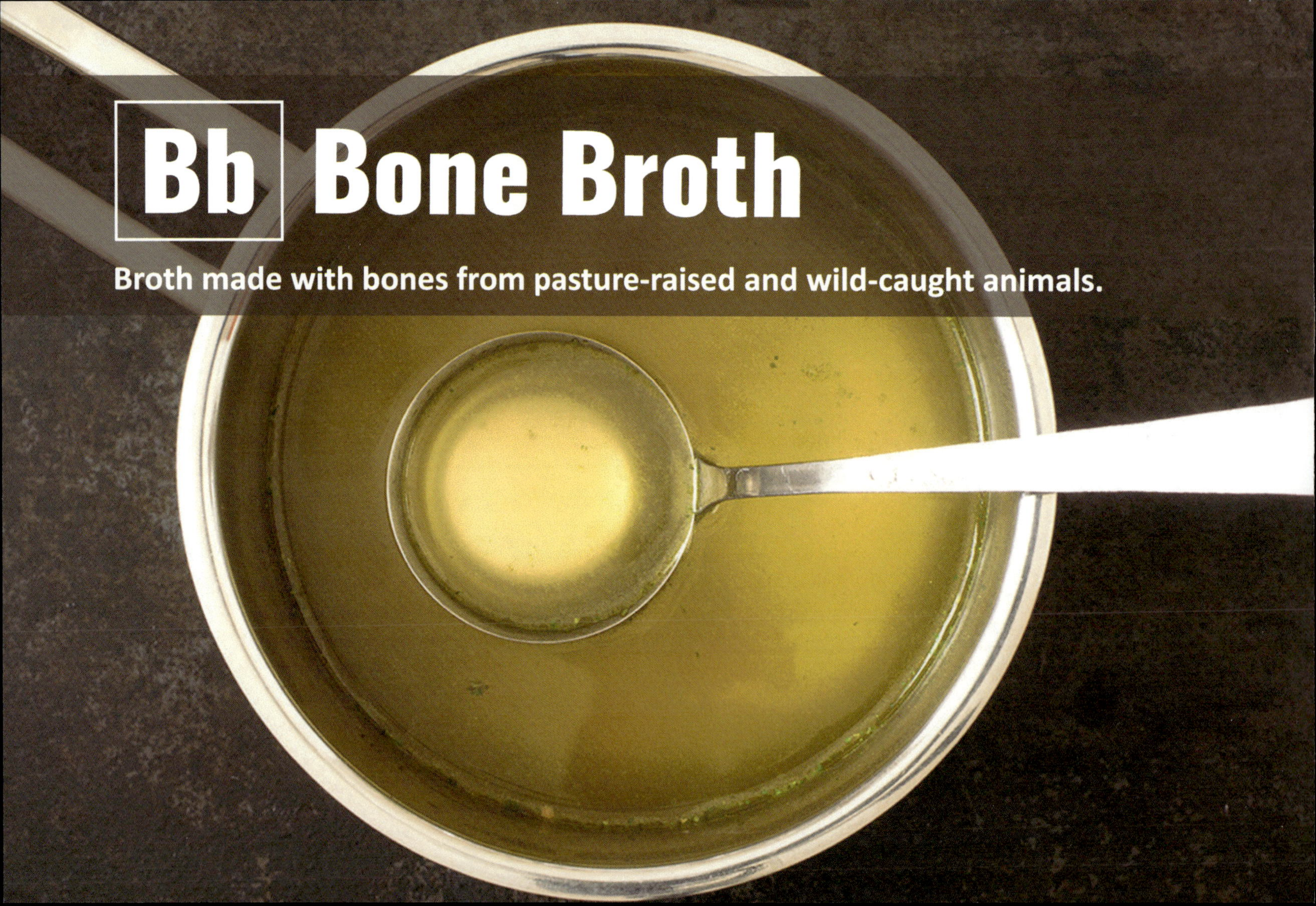

Bb Butter

Raw and cultured butter from cows on pasture is called the "Queen of Fats".

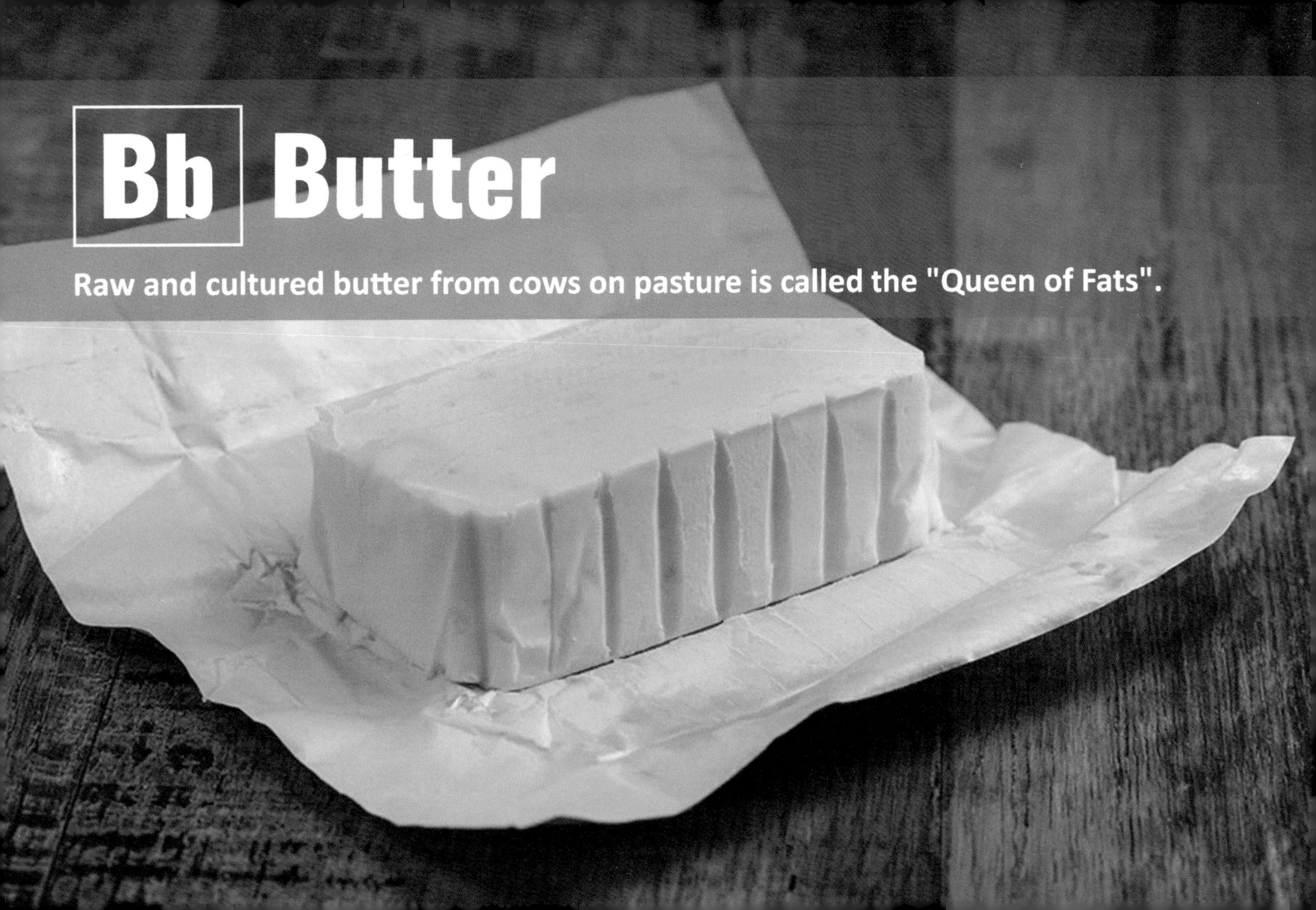

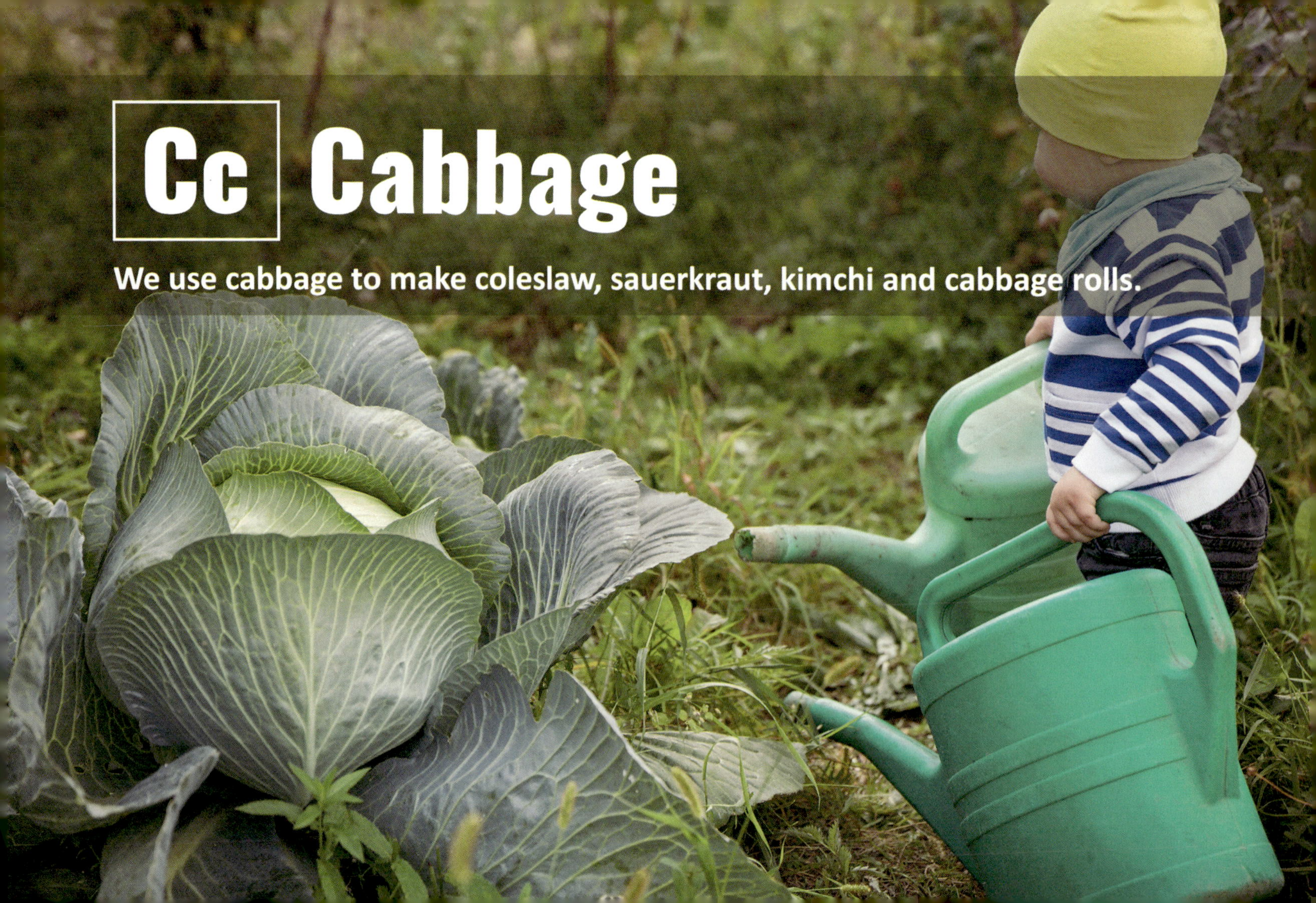

Cc Cabbage

We use cabbage to make coleslaw, sauerkraut, kimchi and cabbage rolls.

Cc Cod Liver Oil

Cod liver oil is a rich source of vitamins A and D, as well as omega-3 fatty acids.

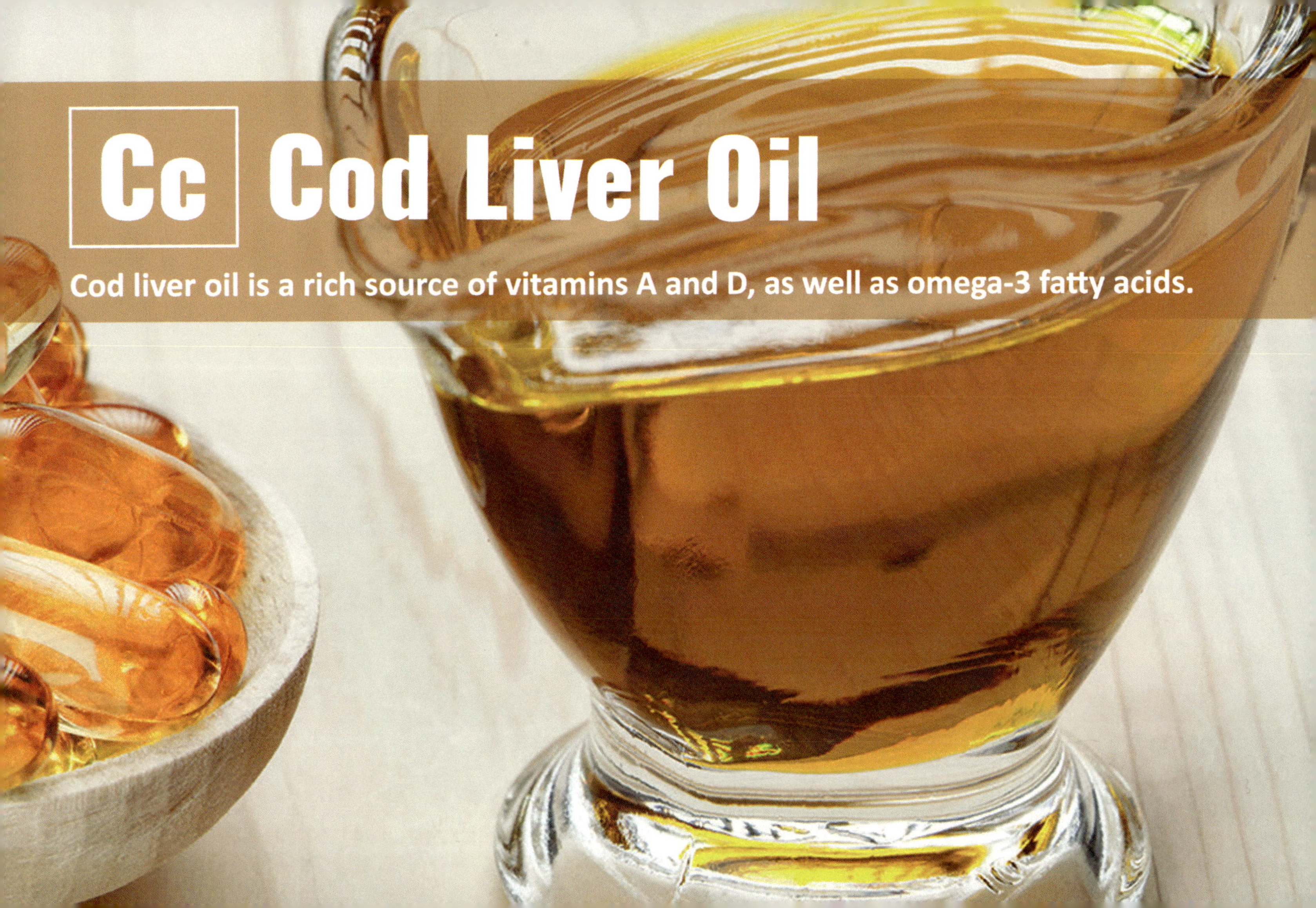

Dd Dairy

Raw and cultured dairy products come from the milk of cows, goats and sheep.

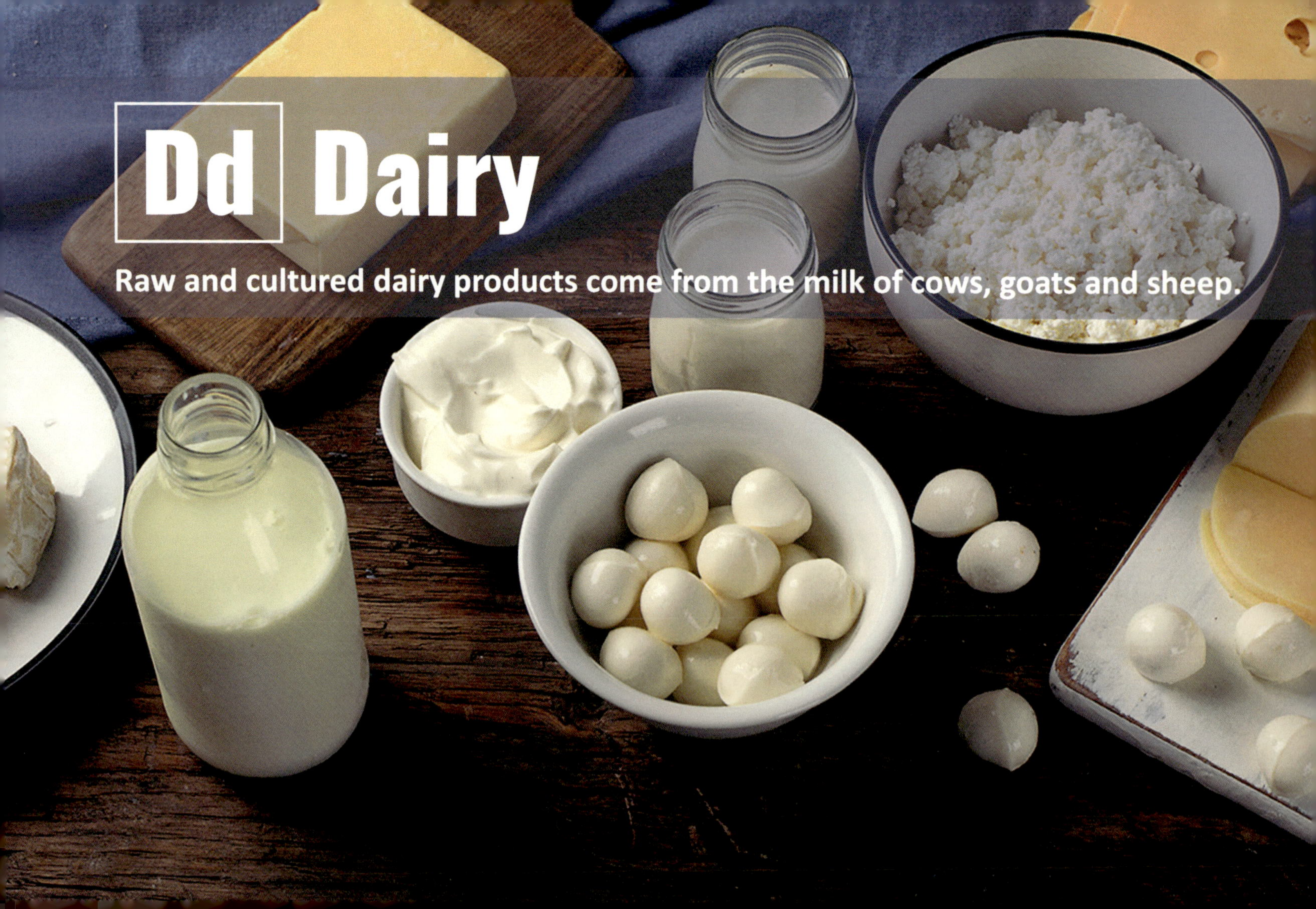

Dd Dates

The date palm tree produces fruit that is dried before we eat them.

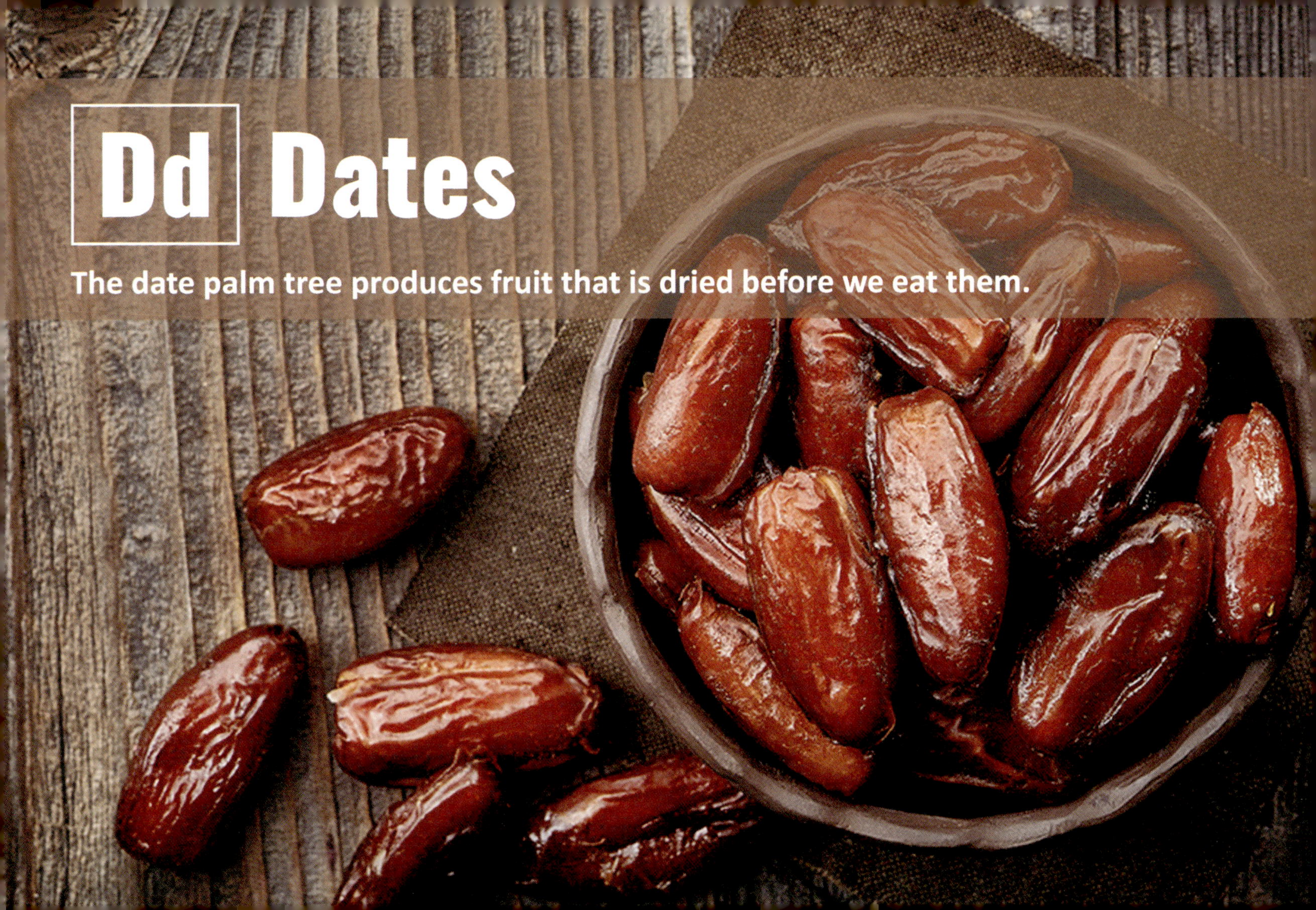

Ee Eggs

Eggs from hens on pasture are described as "nature's perfect food".

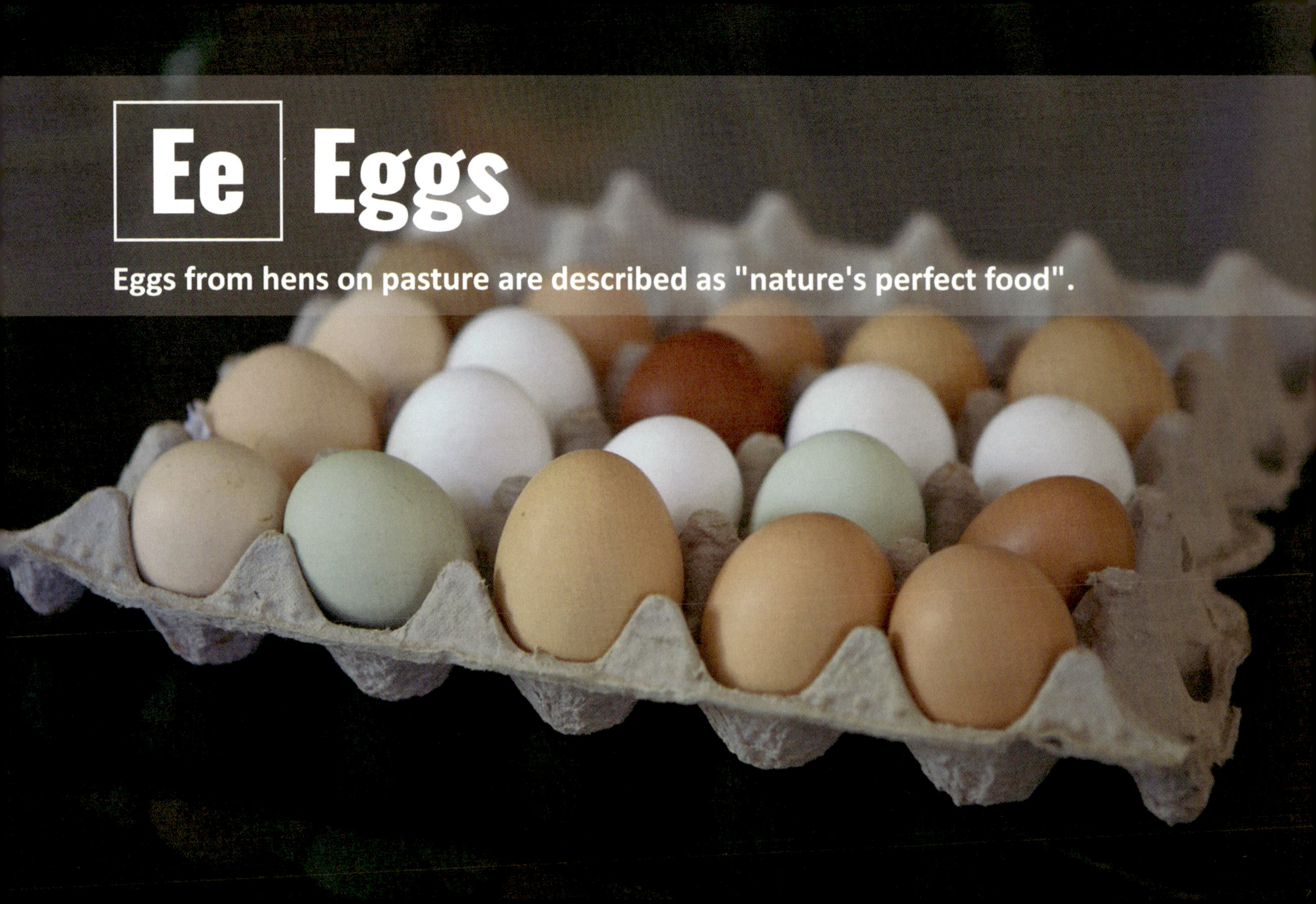

Ee Elderberry

Elderberry syrup can prevent and treat cold or flu symptoms such as a cough.

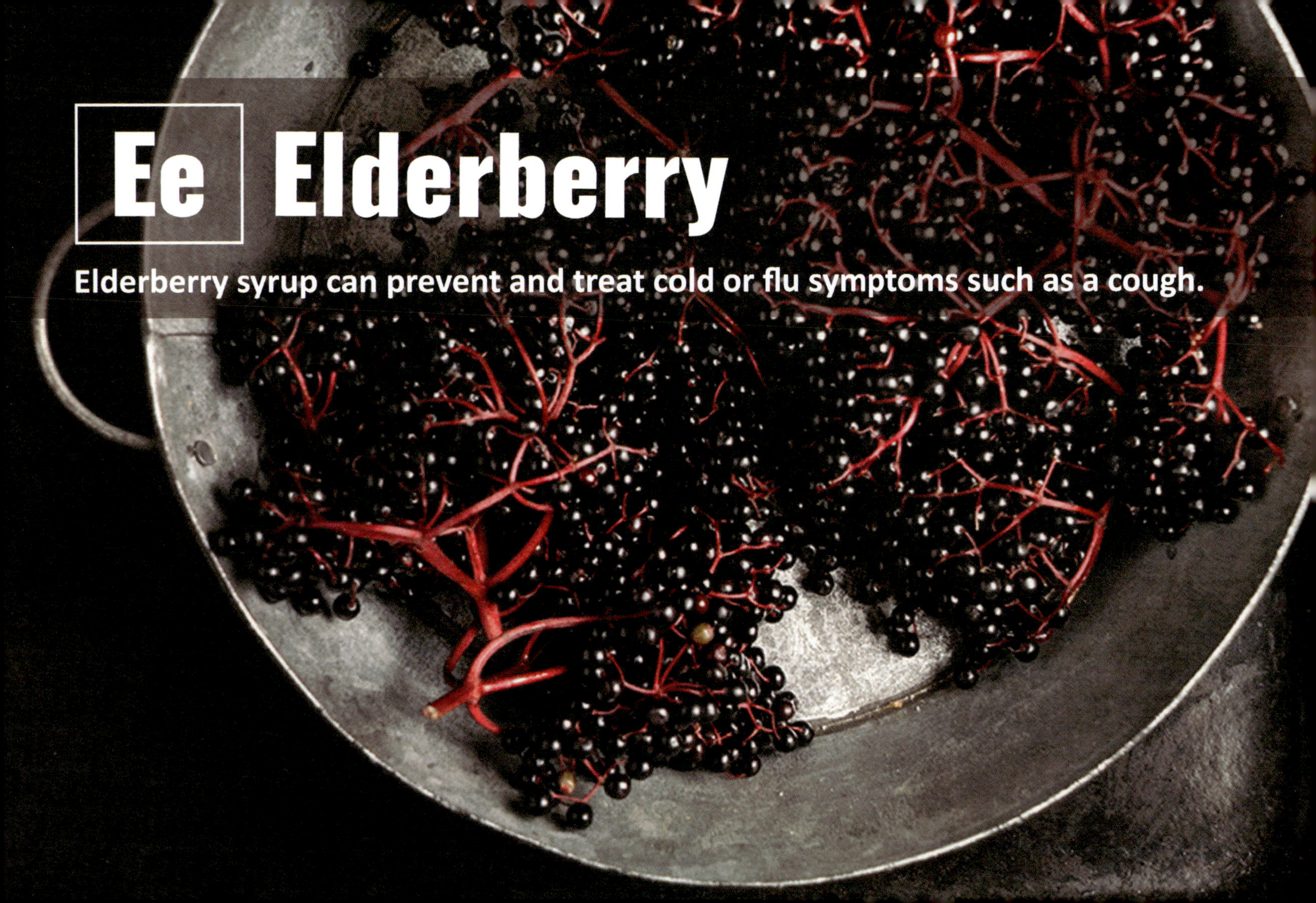

Ff Fat on Fruit

Cultured cream, or crème fraîche, on top of fruit makes it more nutritious.

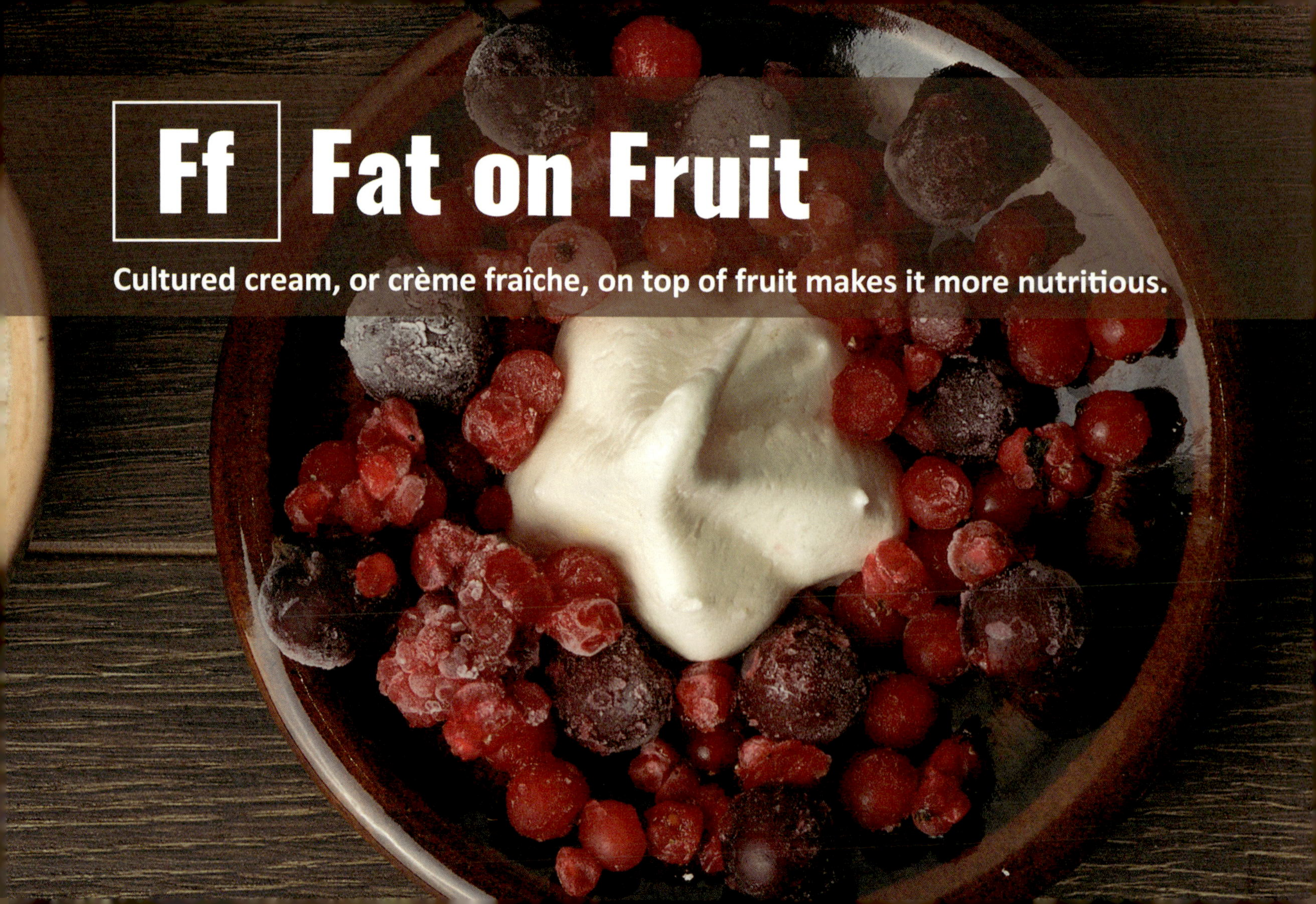

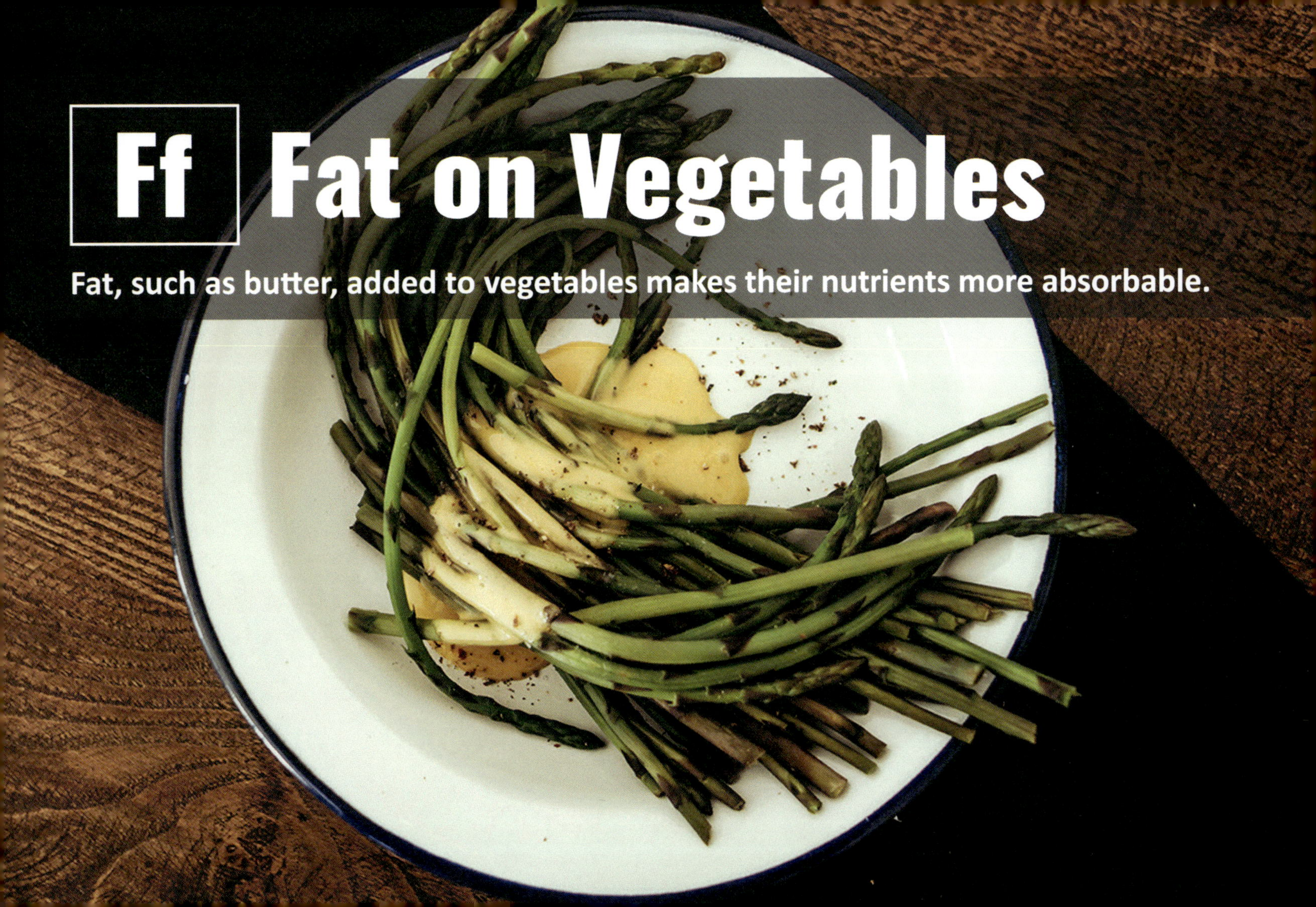

Ff Fat on Vegetables

Fat, such as butter, added to vegetables makes their nutrients more absorbable.

Gg Ghee

Ghee is butter that has had the milk solids removed. It is pure butter fat.

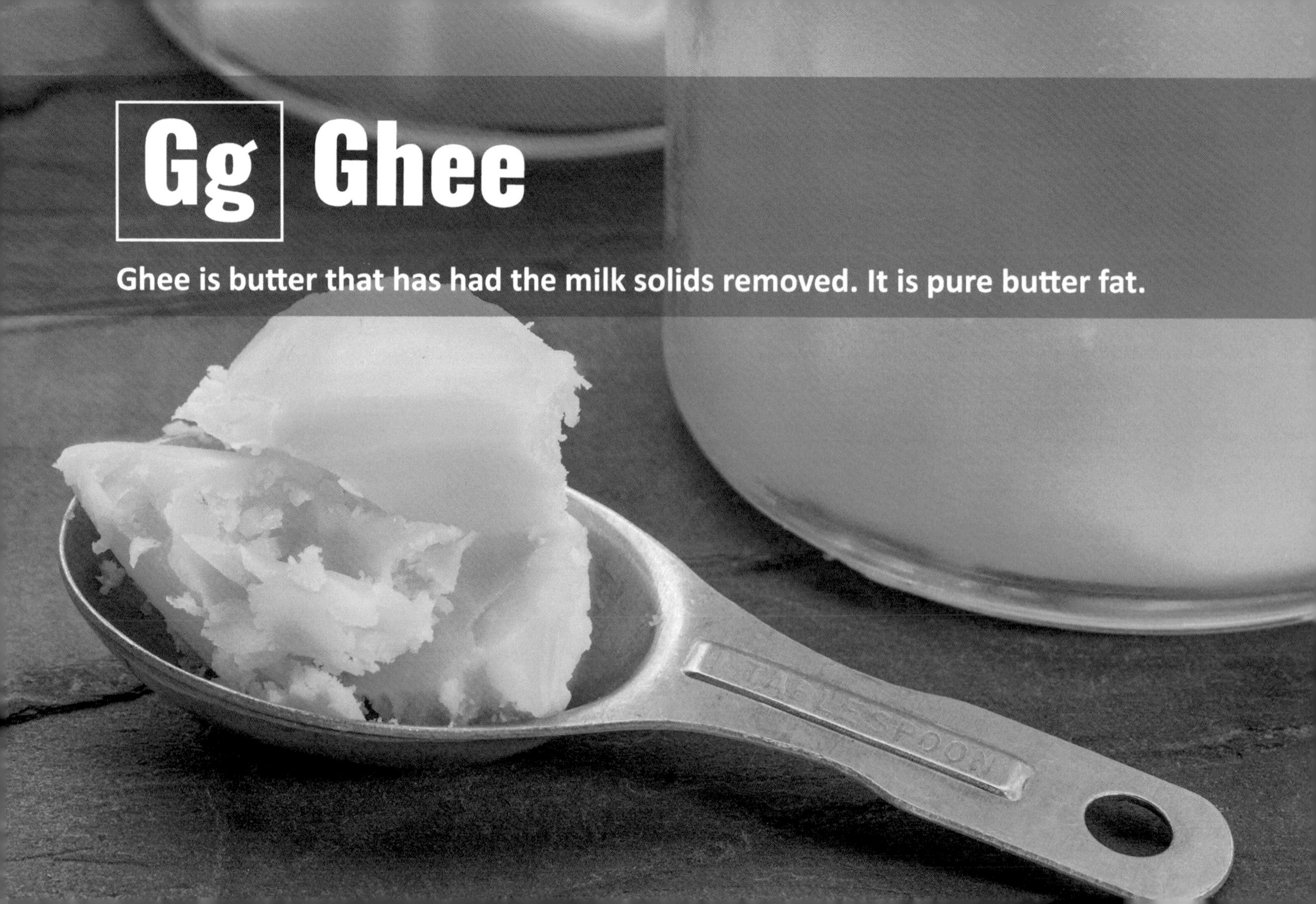

Gg Grass-Fed Meat

This meat comes from animals who only eat their natural diet of pasture and hay.

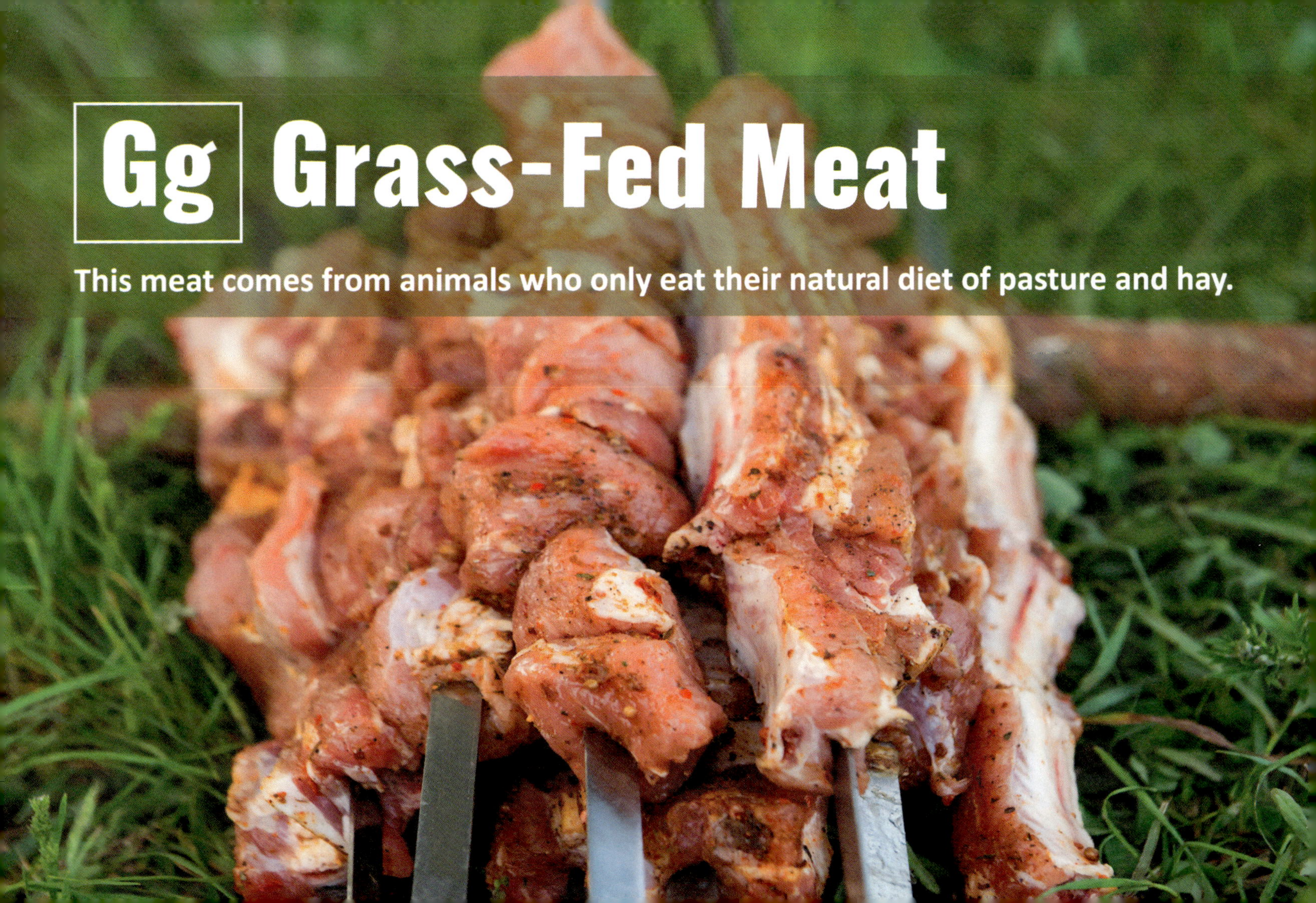

Hh Herbs

Herbs such as mint add flavor and health benefits to the food we prepare.

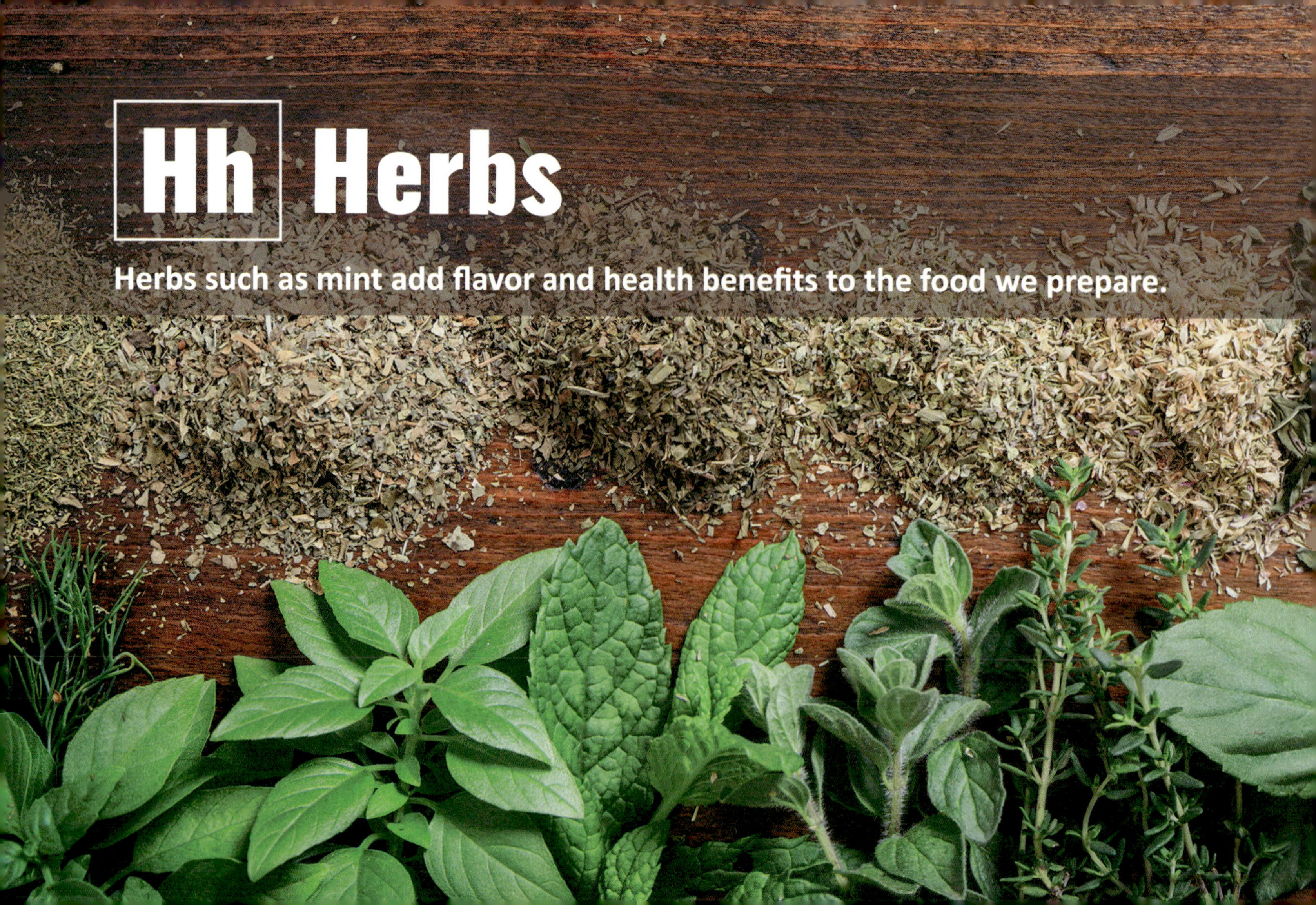

Hh Honey

Bees provide raw, local honey for occasional desserts and sweets.

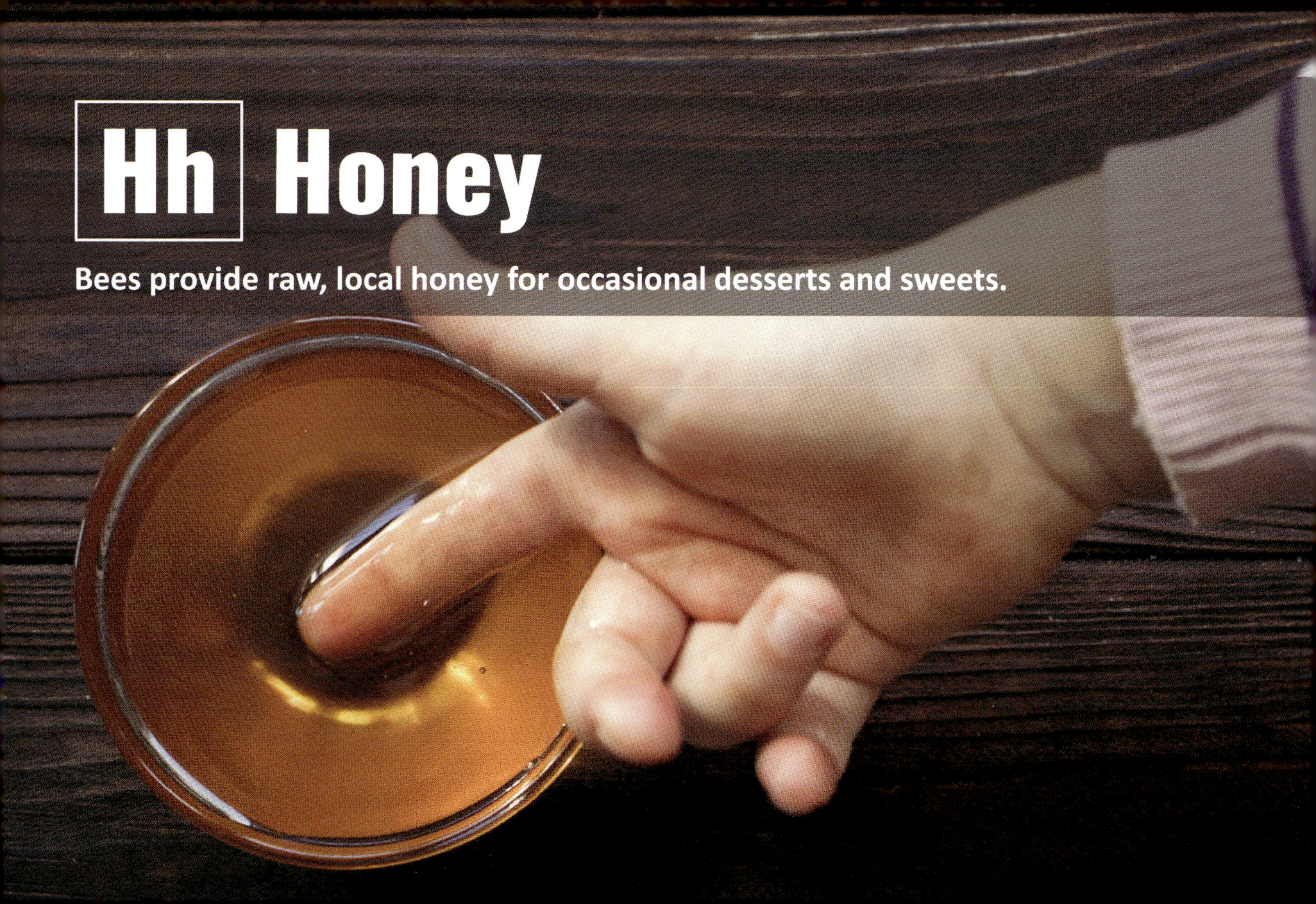

Ii Ice Pop

An ice pop is a water or milk based frozen treat on a stick.

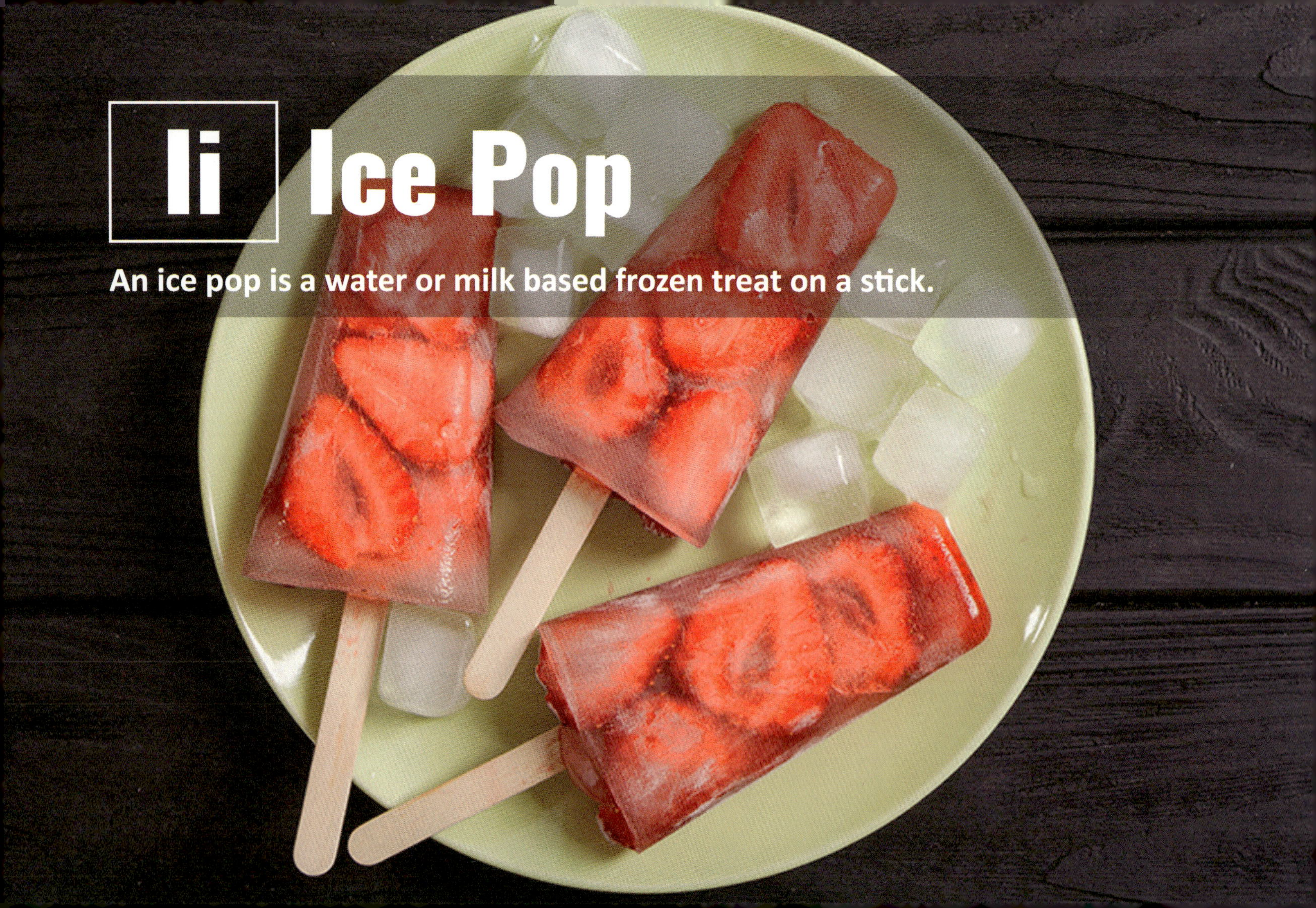

Ii Italian Sausage

It is often described as sausage made of pork and seasoned with fennel or anise.

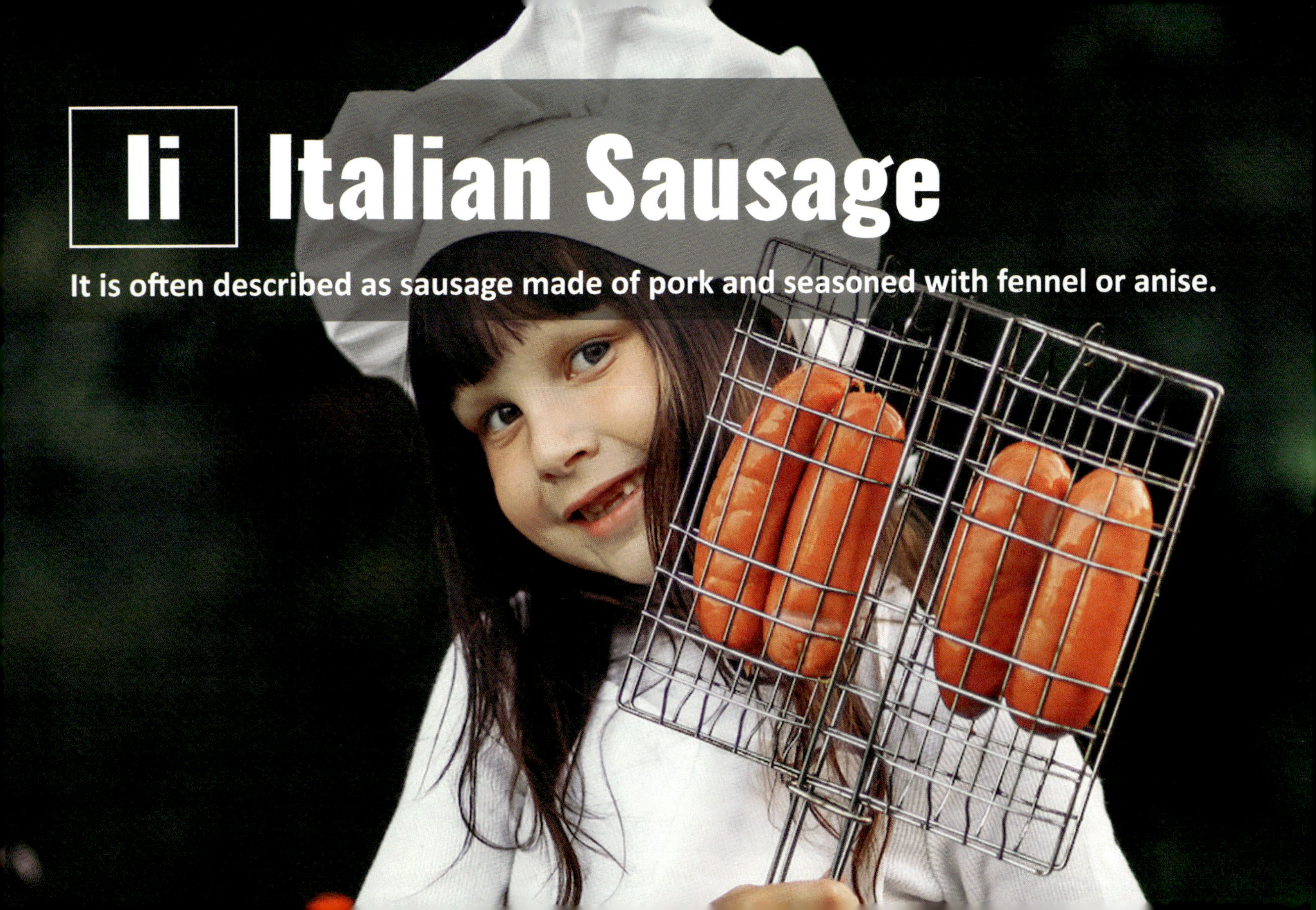

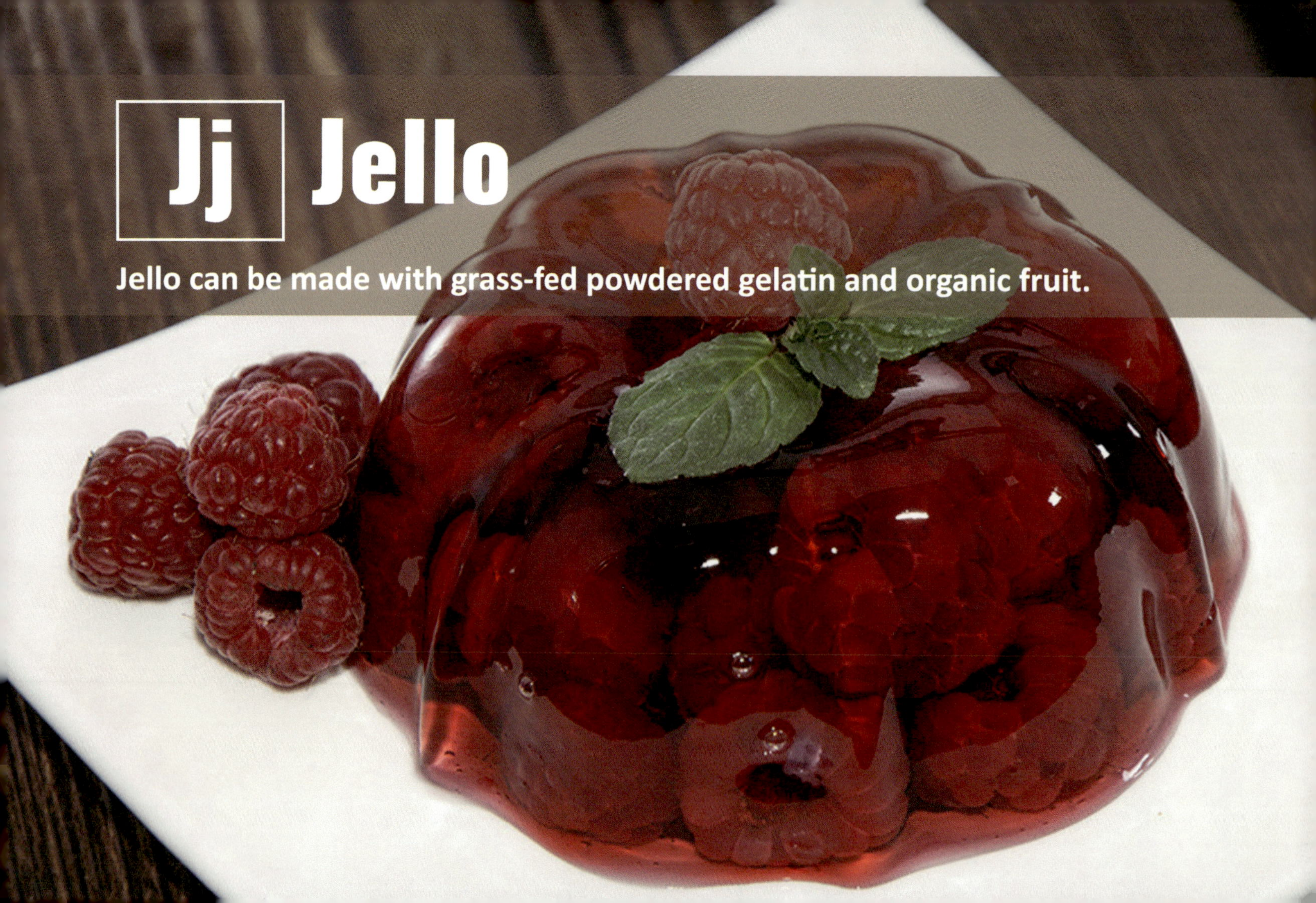

Jj Jello

Jello can be made with grass-fed powdered gelatin and organic fruit.

Jj Jerky

Jerky is meat that has been cut into strips and dried. It's conveninet for travel!

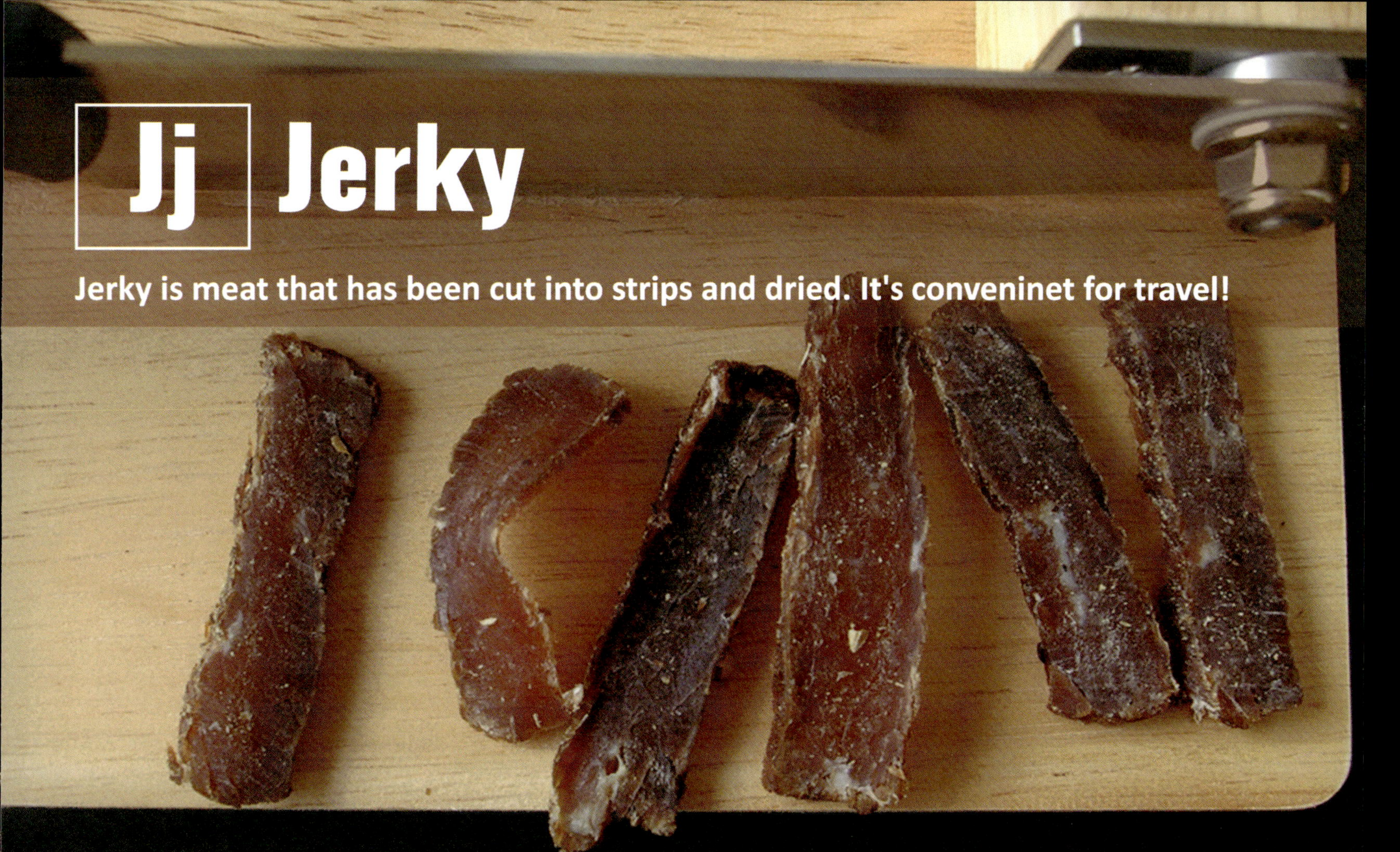

Kk Kefir

Kefir grains are used to ferment, or sour, raw milk.

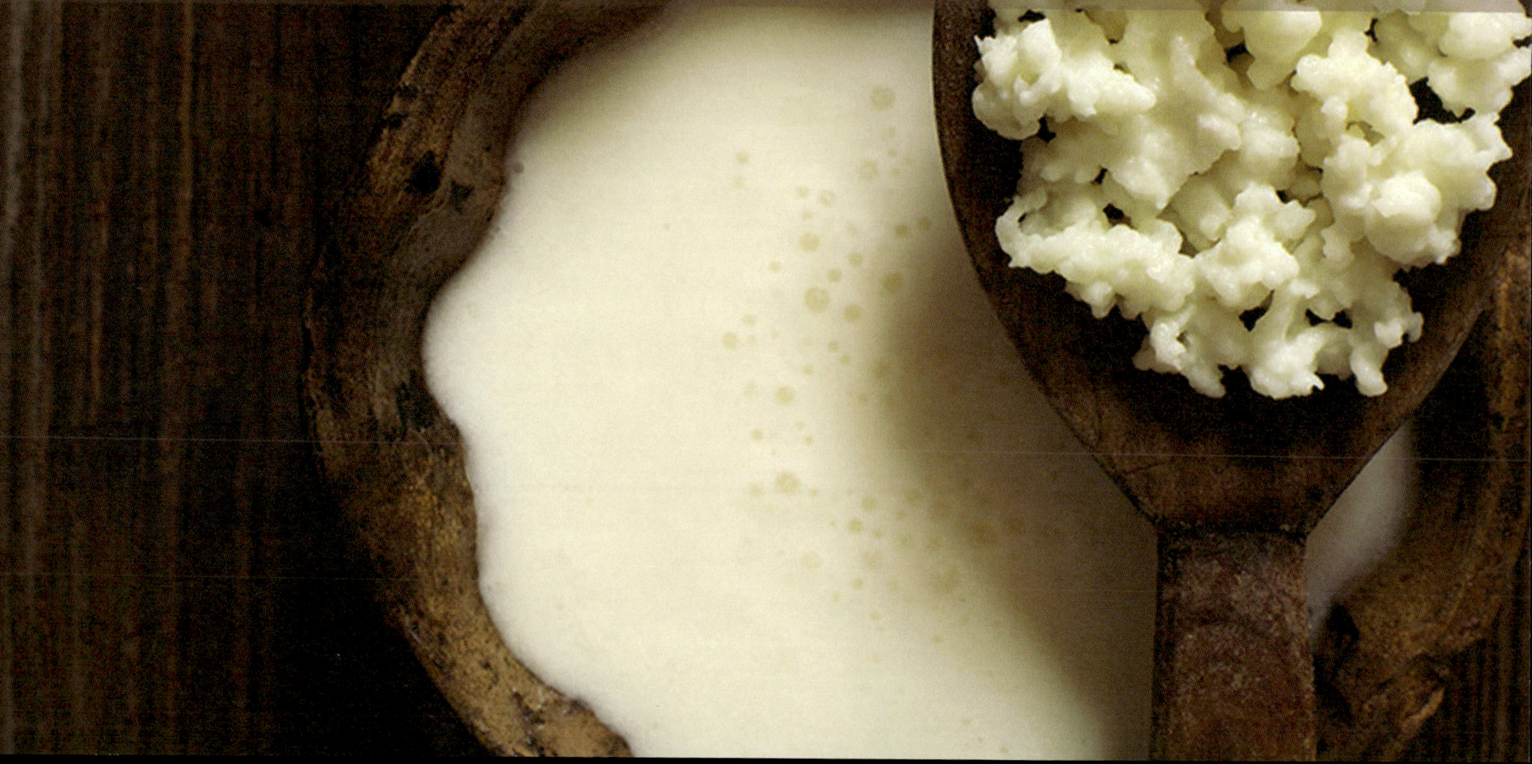

Kk Kombucha

A beverage made by fermenting sweet tea with a culture of yeast and bacteria.

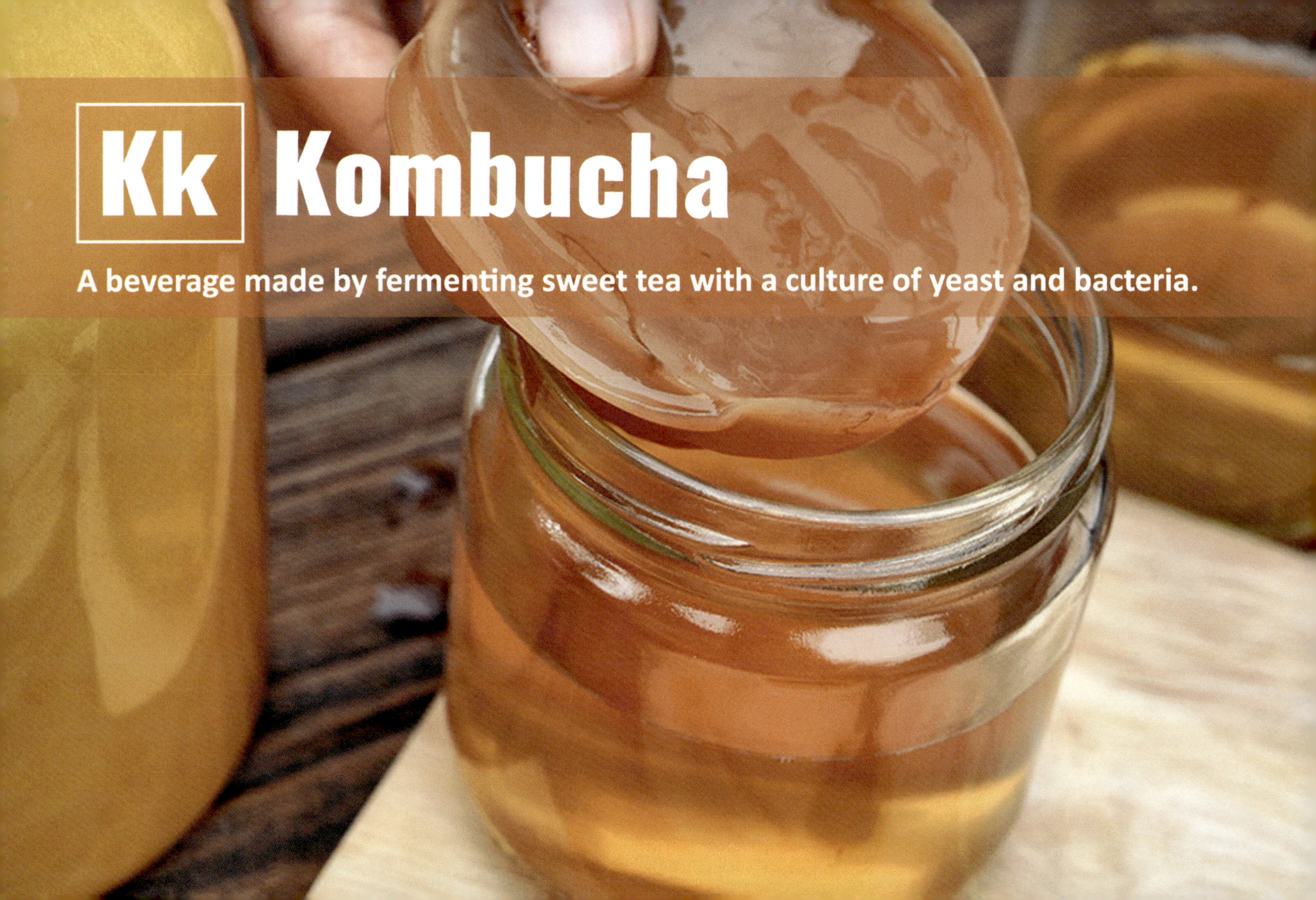

Ll Lard

Lard from pastured pigs is a traditional fat. It is very high in vitamin D.

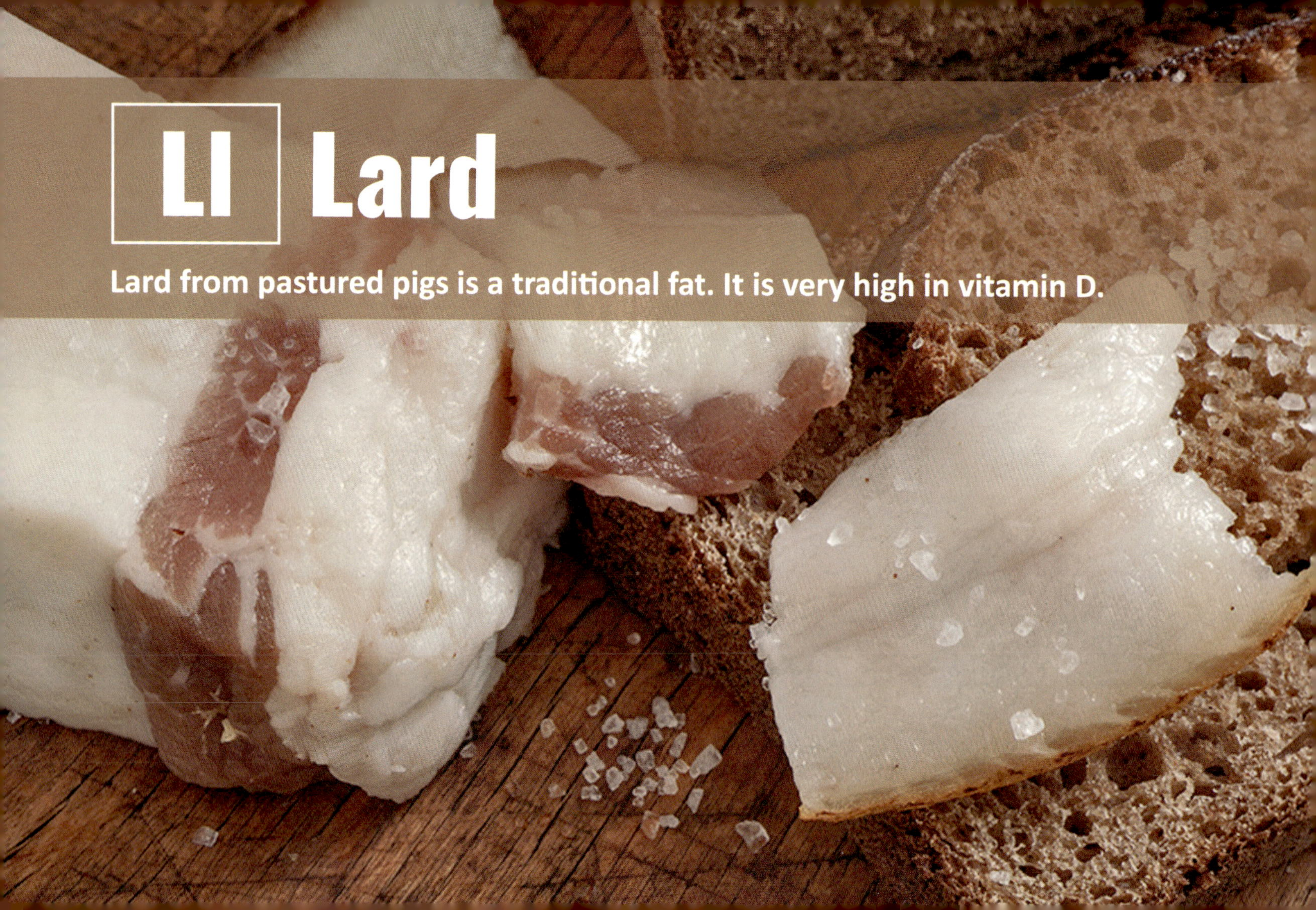

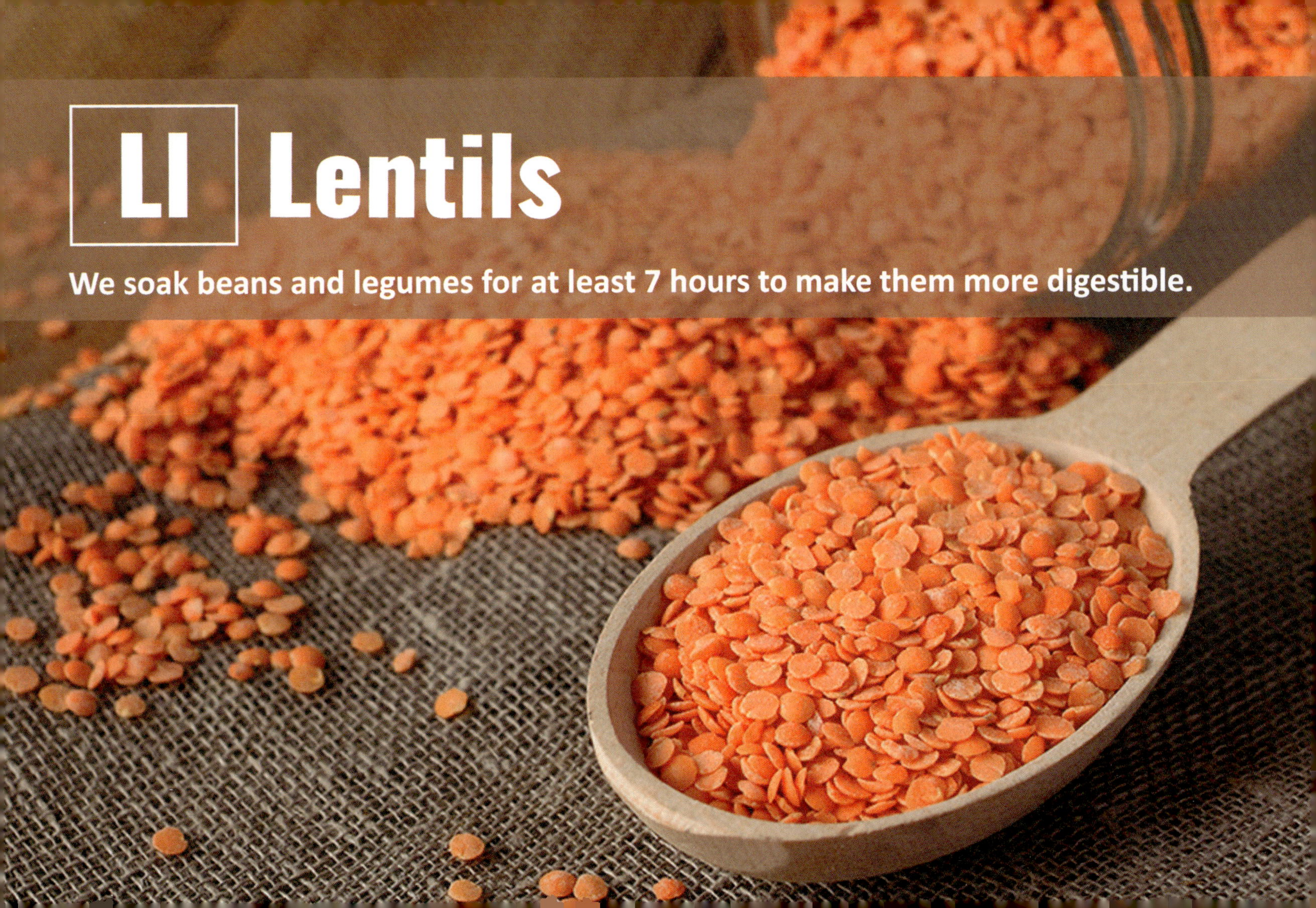
LI
Lentils
We soak beans and legumes for at least 7 hours to make them more digestible.

Mm Mayonnaise

Homemade mayonnaise is made with raw egg yolks from hens on pasture.

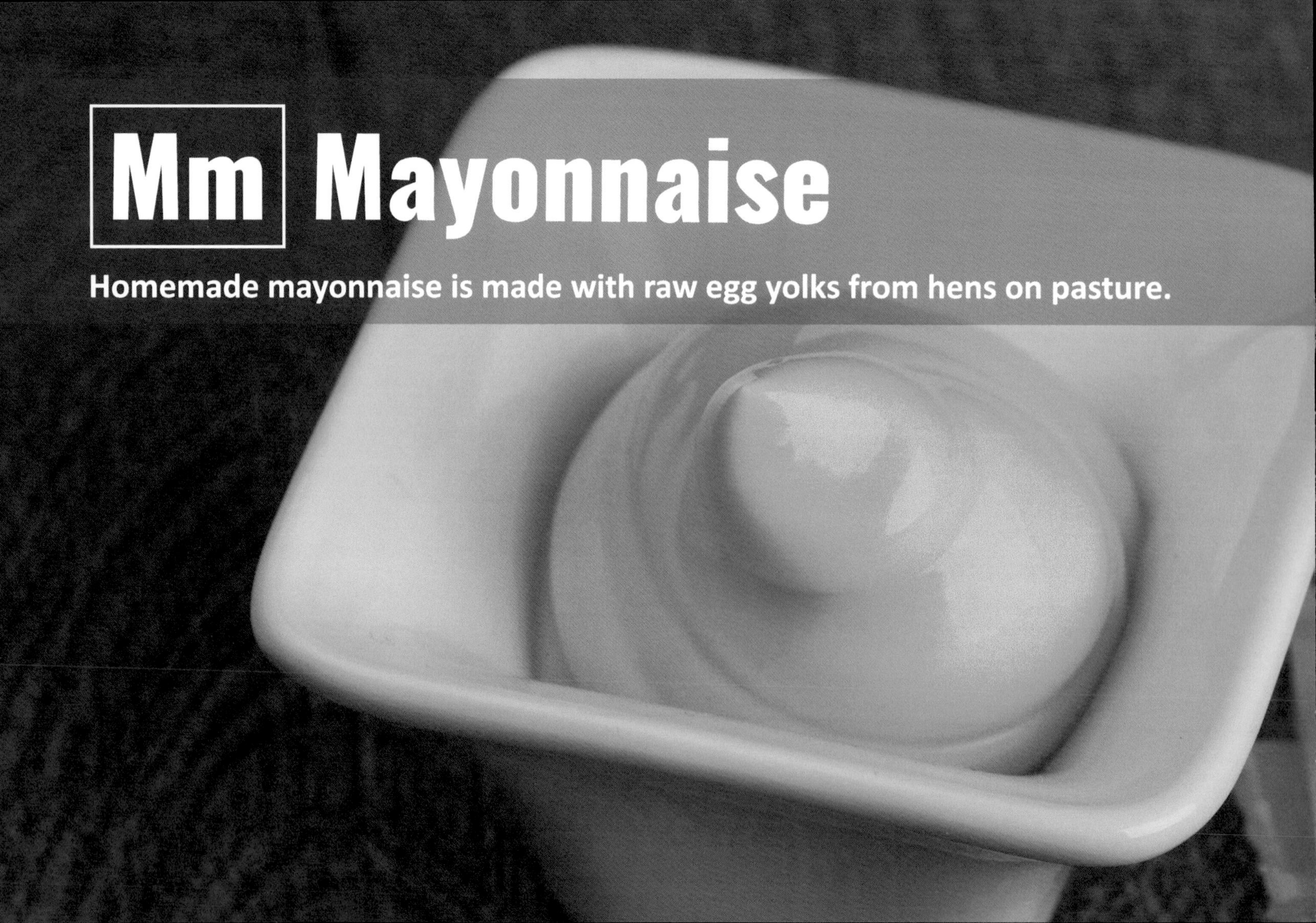

Mm Milk

Raw milk, from grazing animals, is not pasteurized or homogenized.

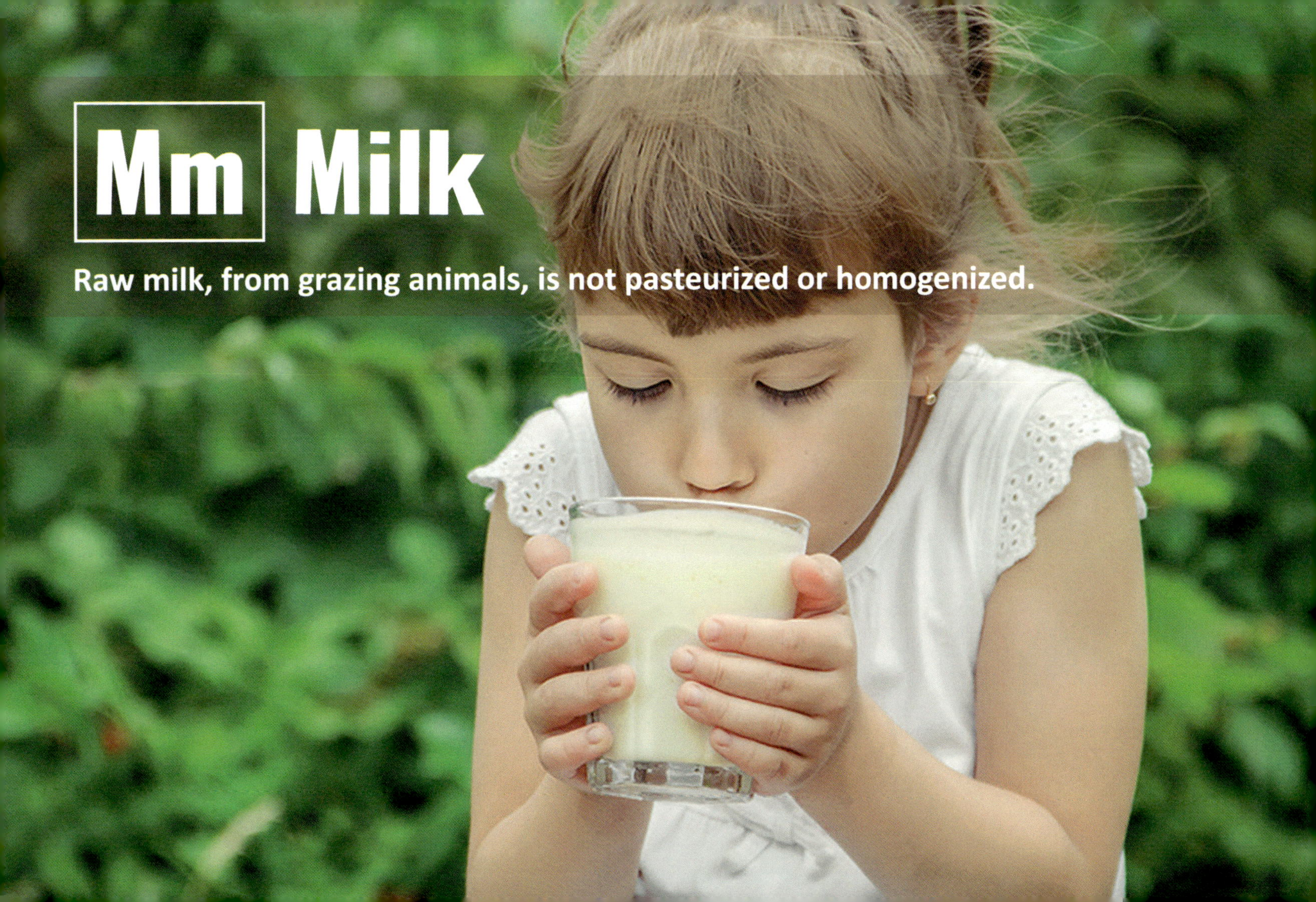

Nn Nattō

Nattō is a traditional Japanese dish made from fermented soybeans.

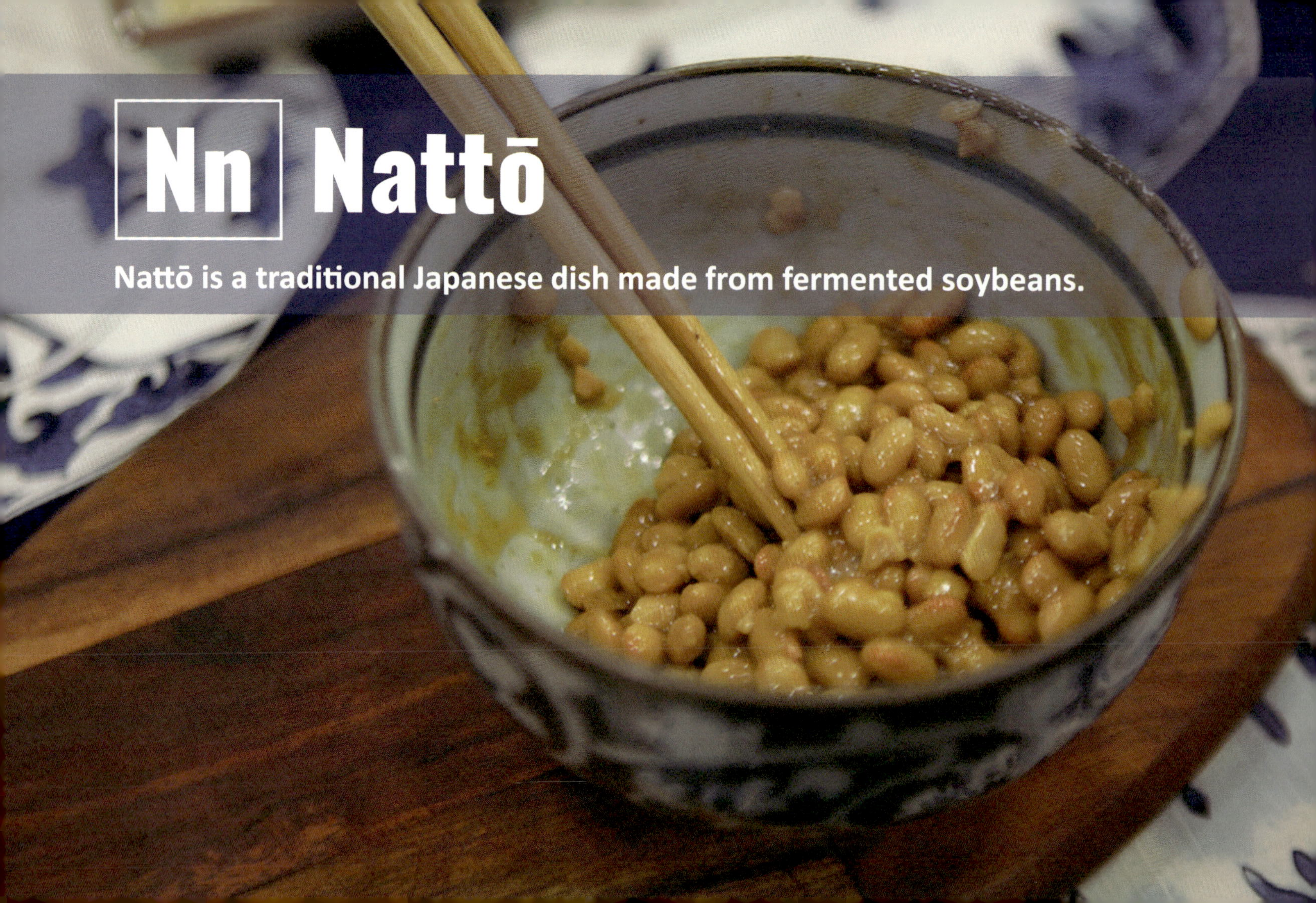

Nn Nori

Nori is the Japanese name for seaweed. It is a sea vegetable that we can eat.

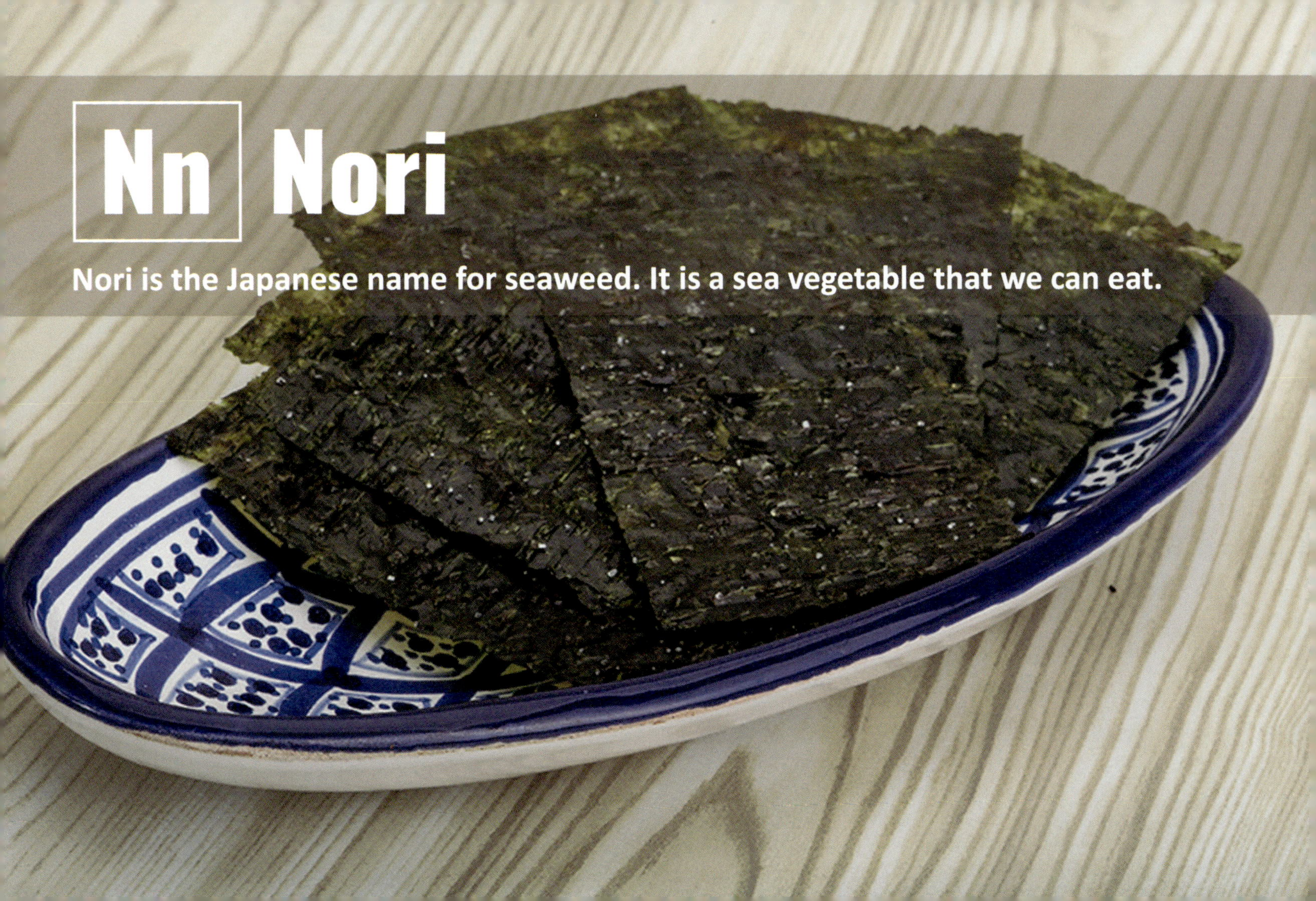

Oo Oatmeal

We soak oats overnight in lemon juice, yogurt or whey before cooking them.

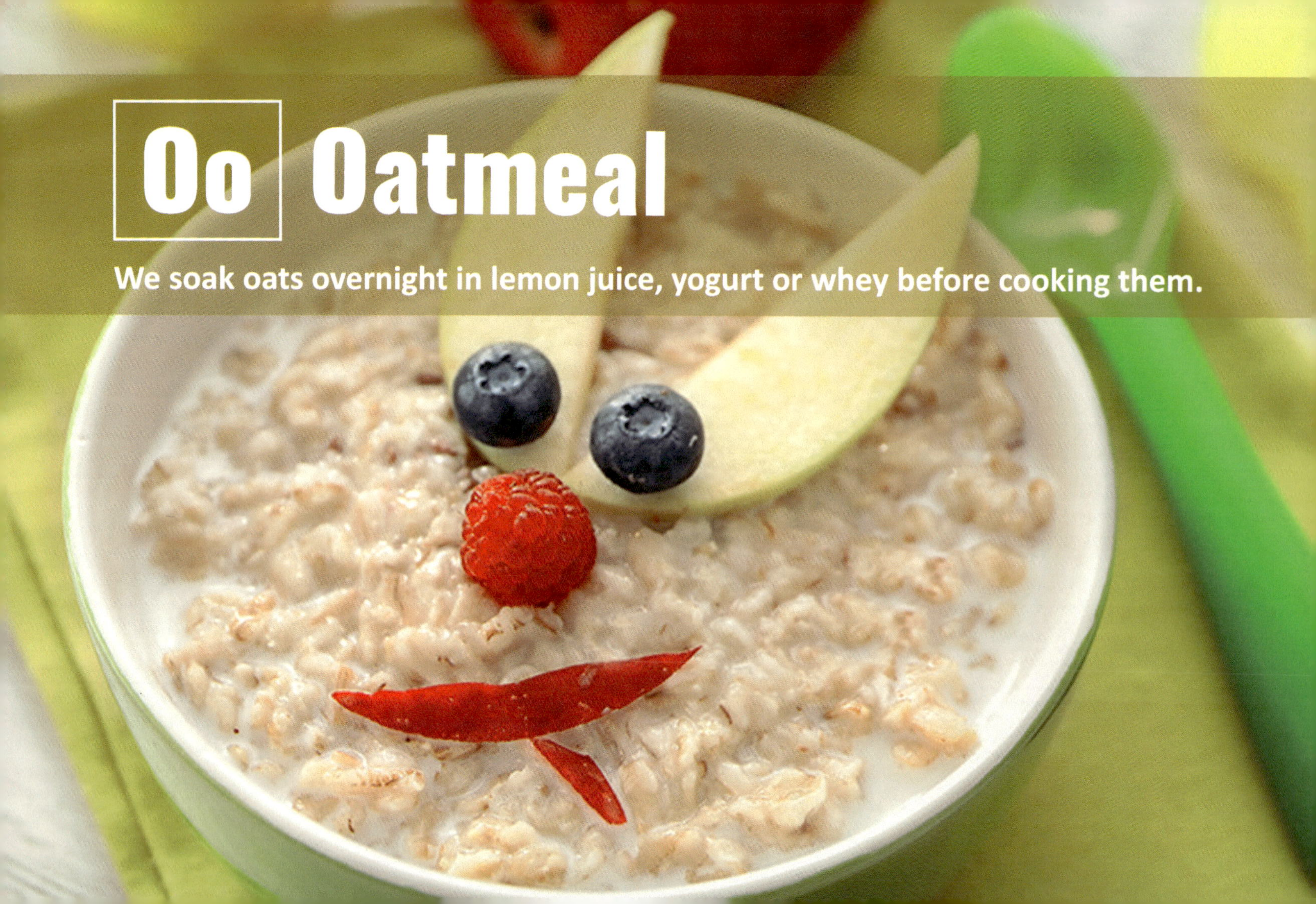

Oo Organ Meats

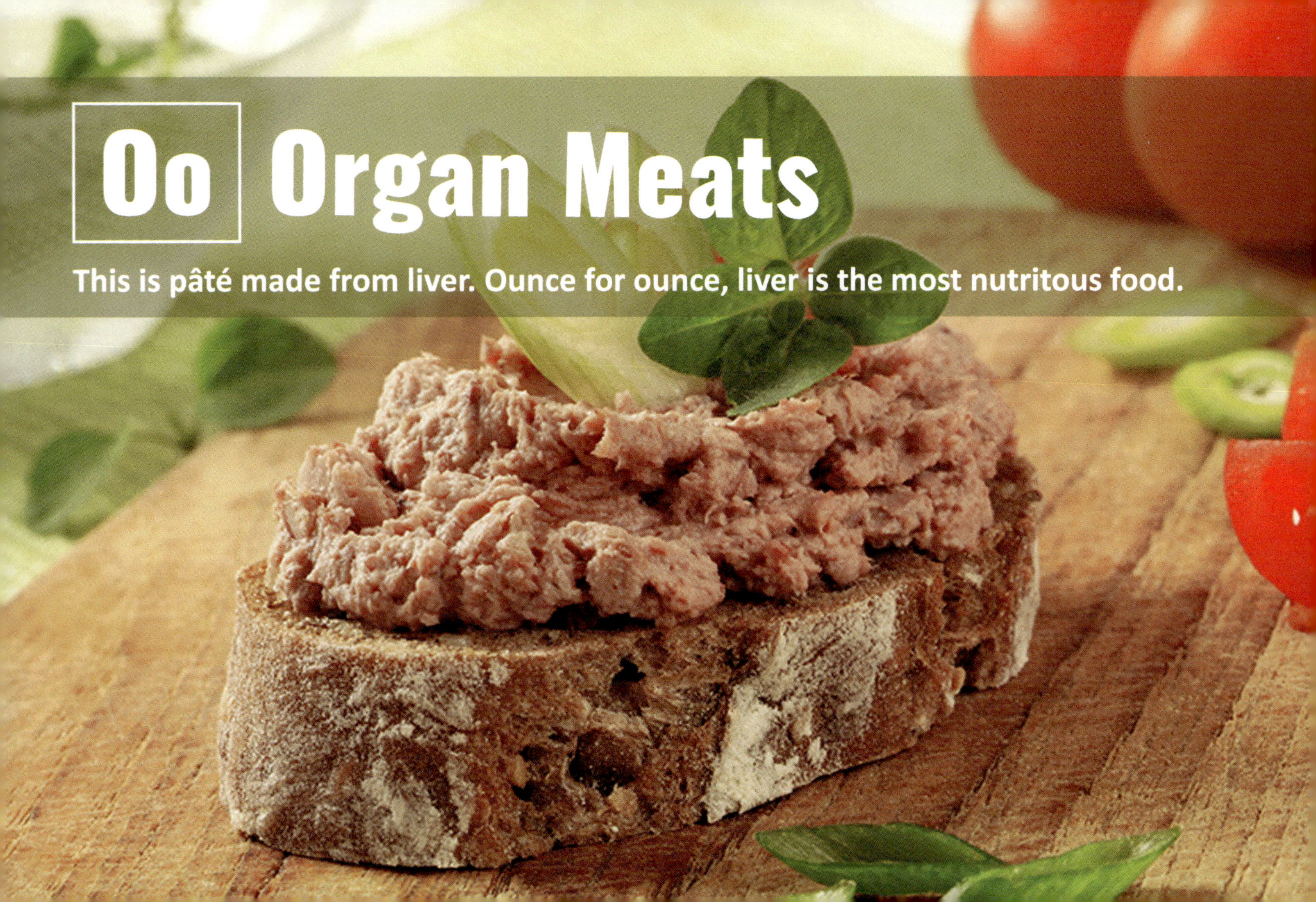

This is pâté made from liver. Ounce for ounce, liver is the most nutritous food.

Pp Pastured Poultry

Pastured chickens forage for wild seeds, worms, insects and other animal foods.

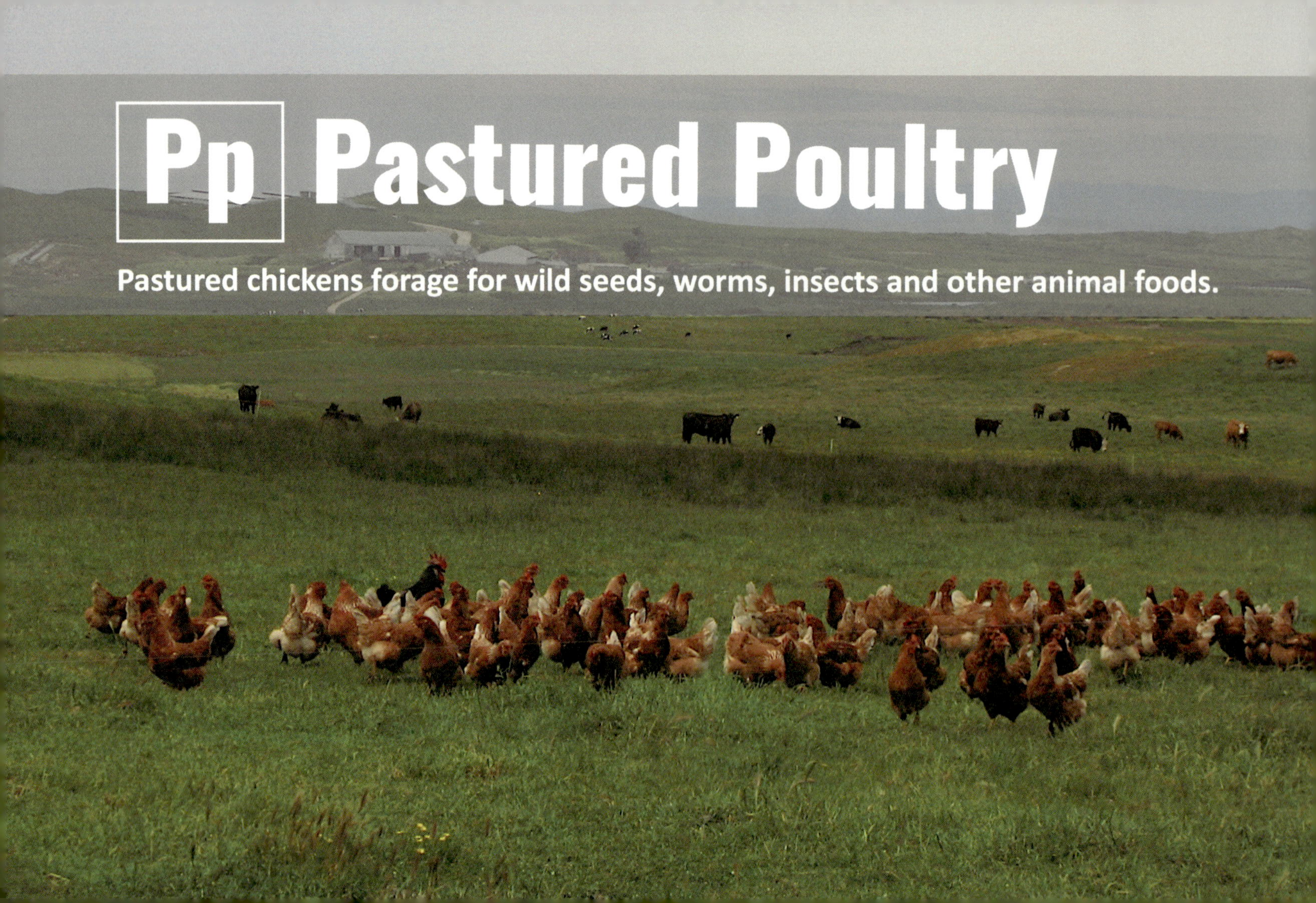

Pp Pickles

Pickling cucumbers need to be fermented in water and sea salt to make pickles.

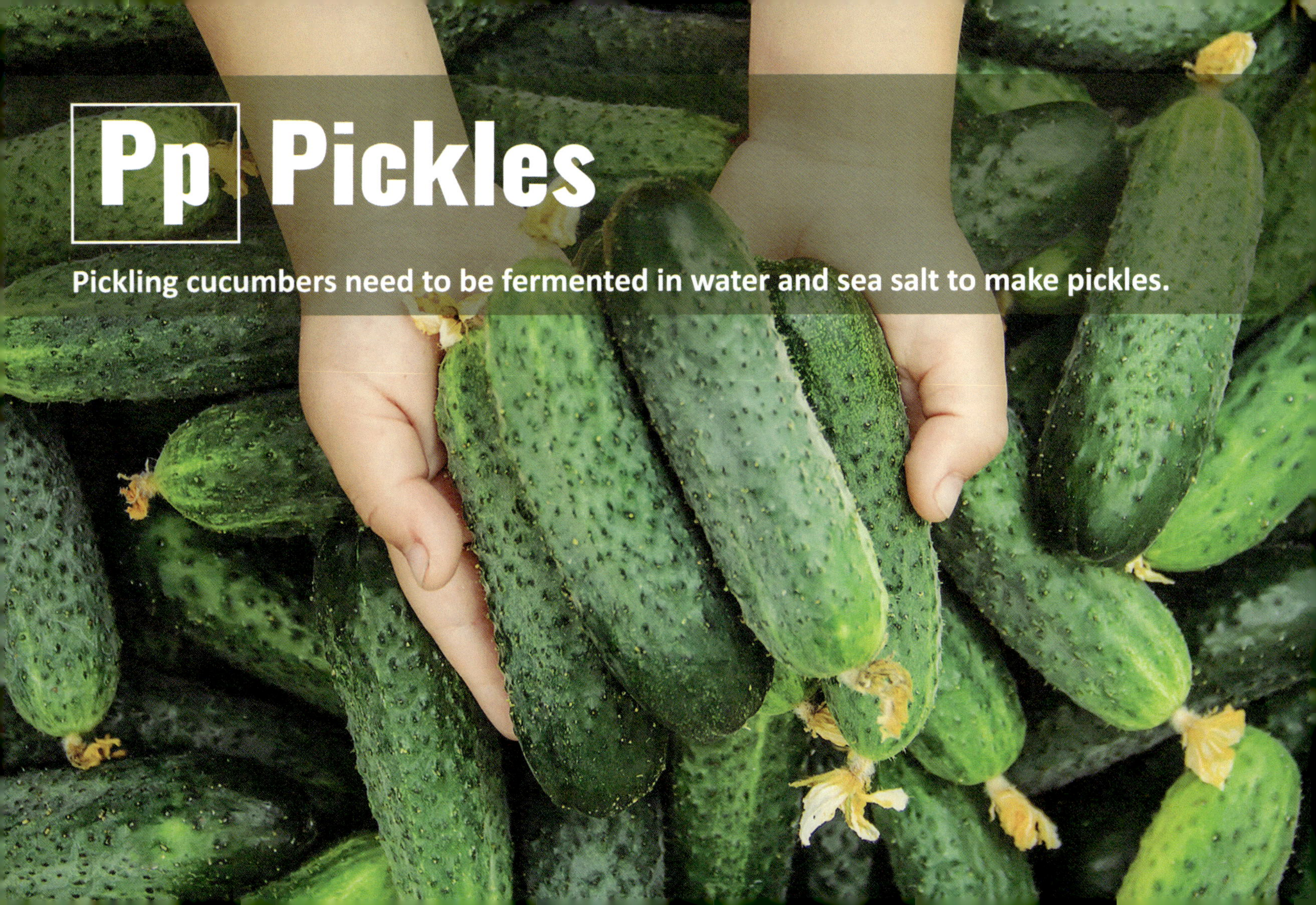

Qq Quail

These spotted eggs come from a female quail; a type of game bird.

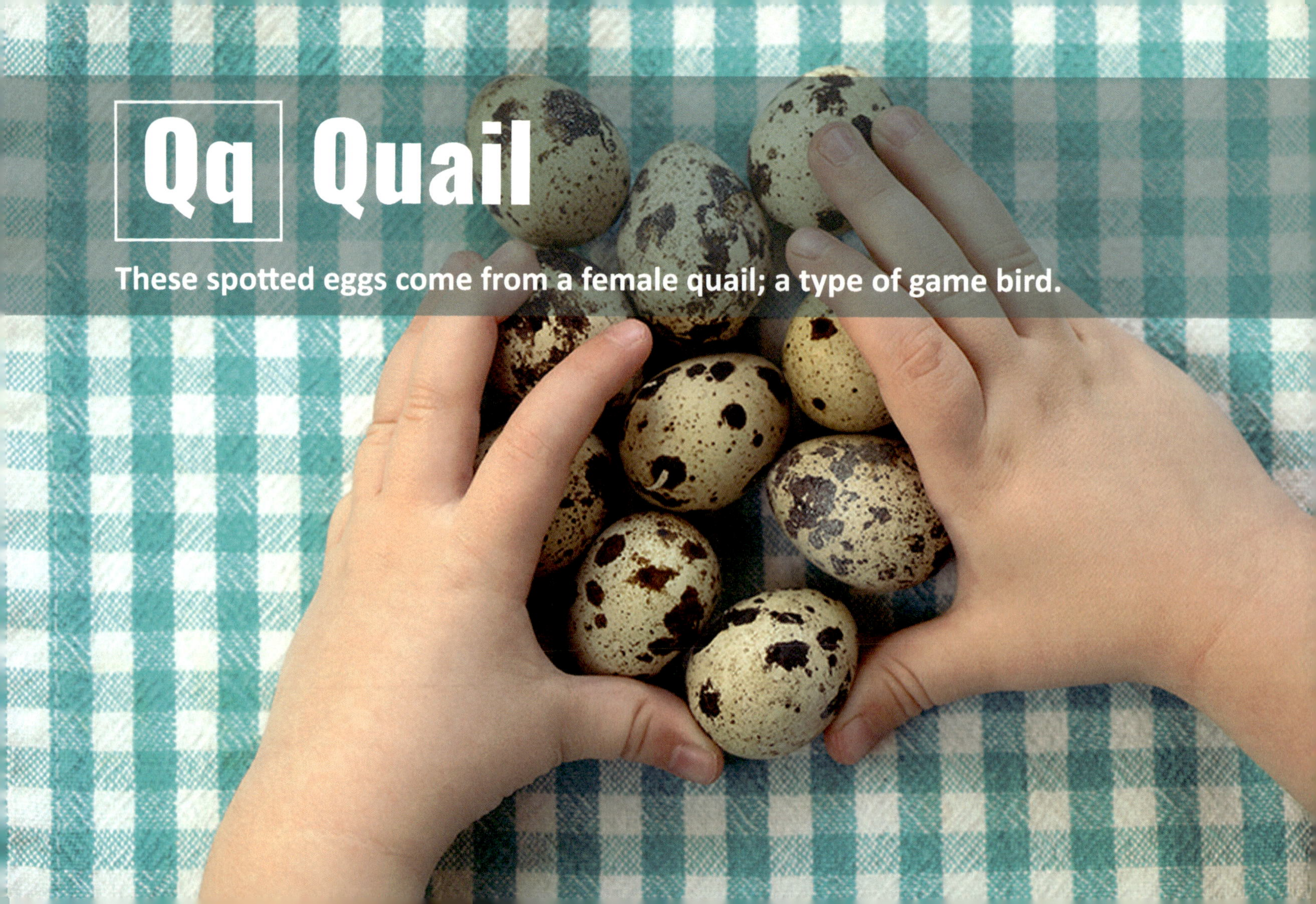

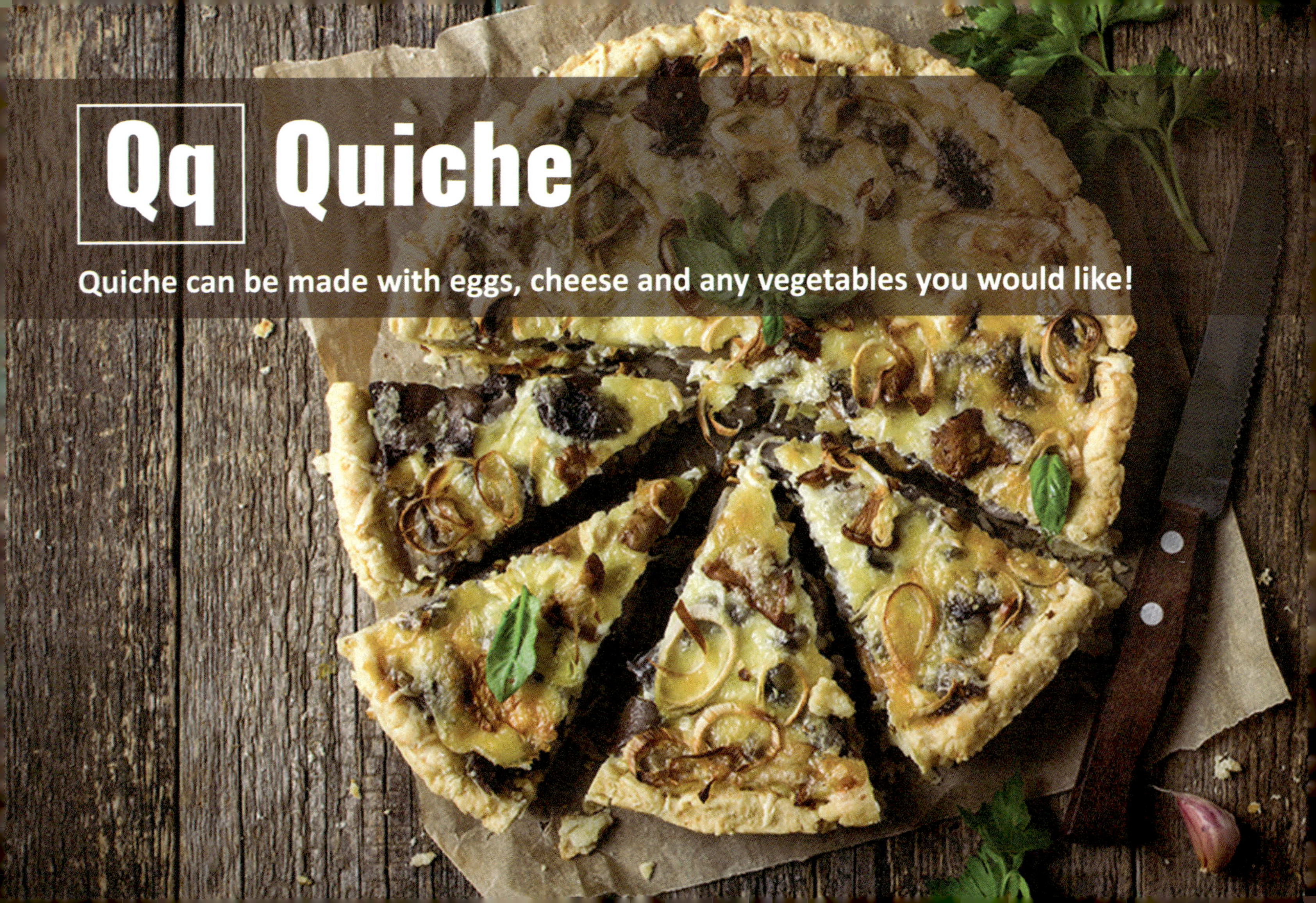

Qq Quiche

Quiche can be made with eggs, cheese and any vegetables you would like!

Rr Raw Oysters

These oysters first need to be shucked, or opened, in order to eat them!

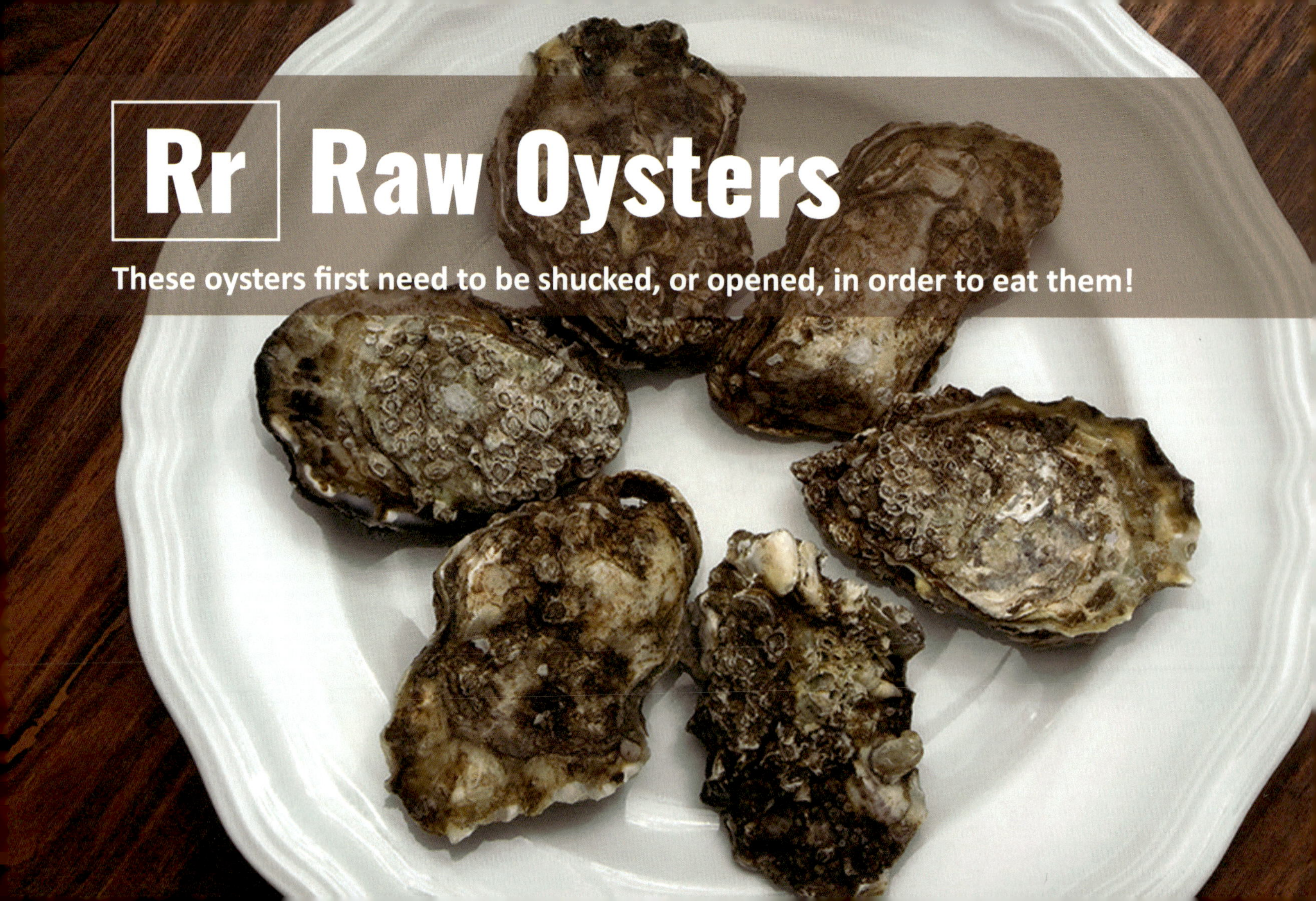

Rr Roe

These are the eggs from a female salmon fish. They are also called cavier.

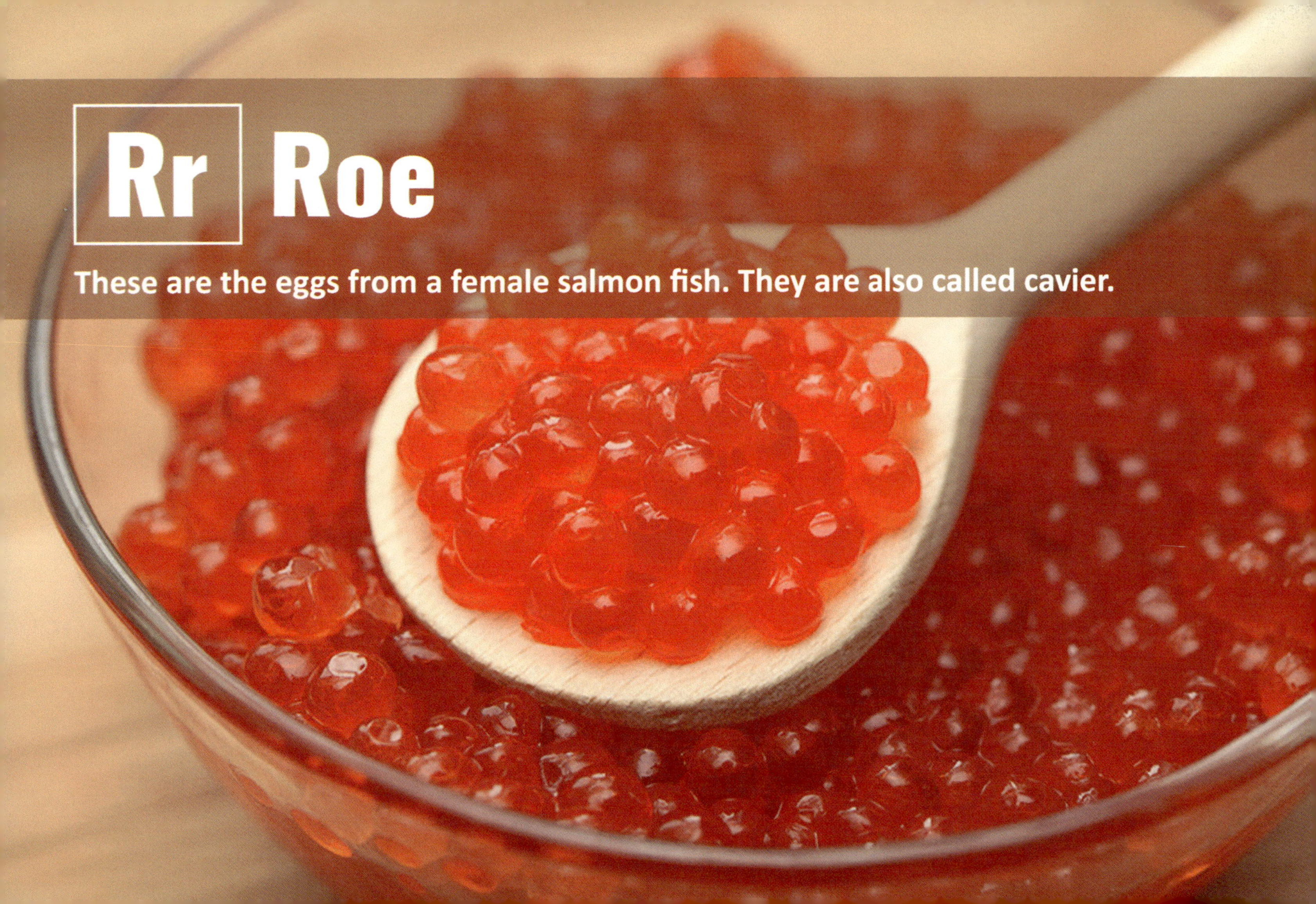

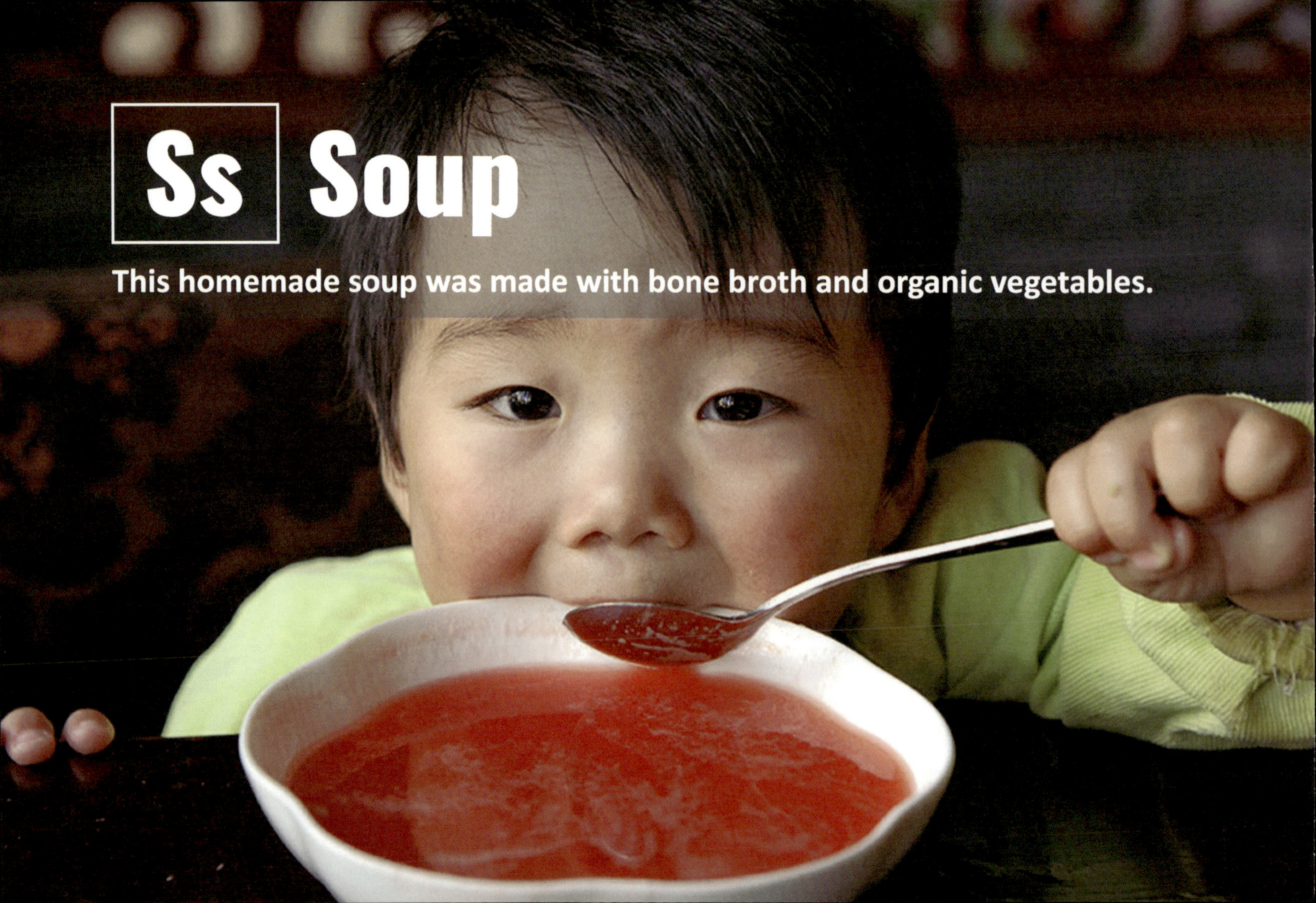

Ss Soup

This homemade soup was made with bone broth and organic vegetables.

Ss Sourdough

Sourdough bread is made with fermented grains that are easier for us to disgest.

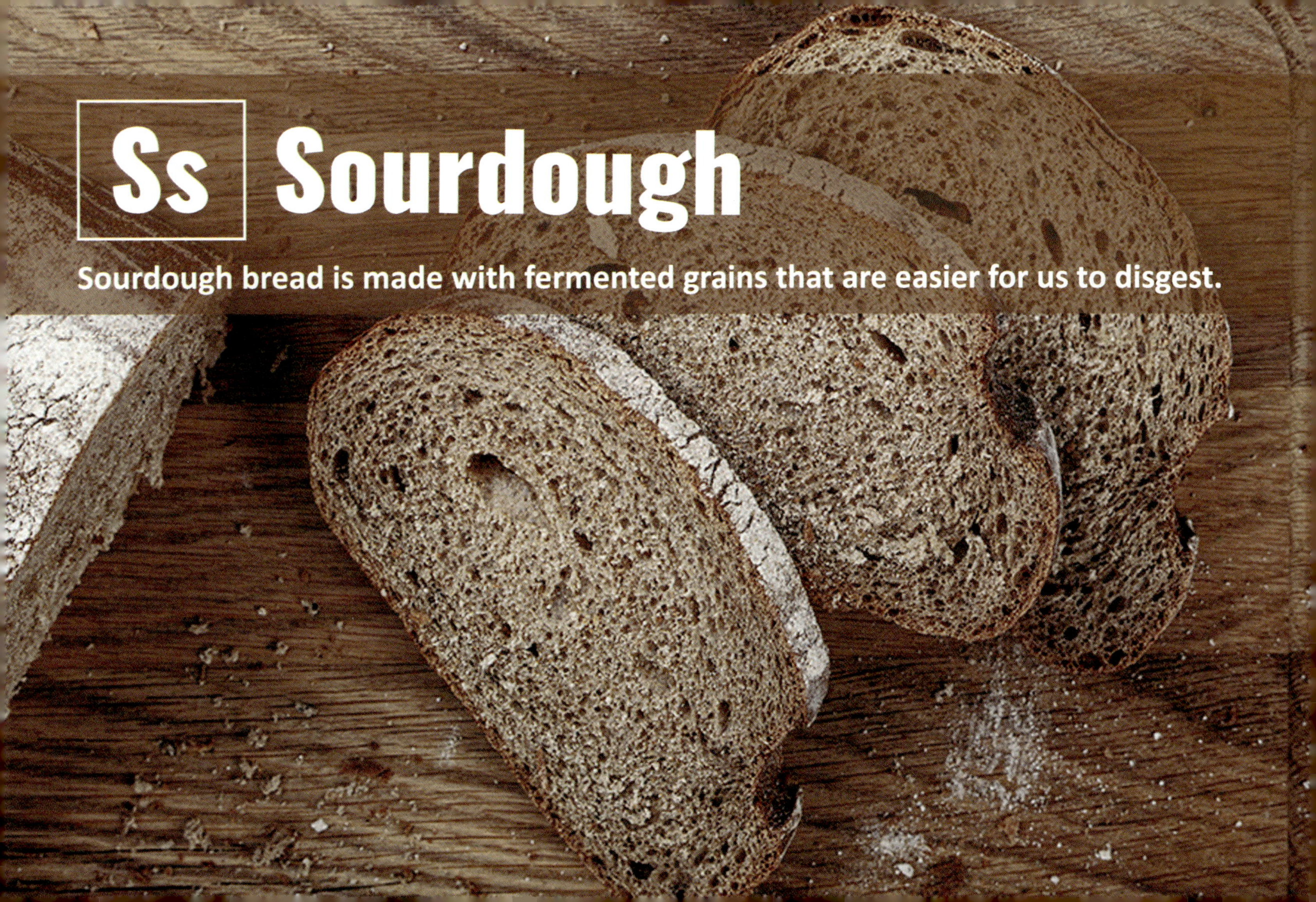

Tt Tongue

We eat the entire animal from nose to tail! This is beef tongue.

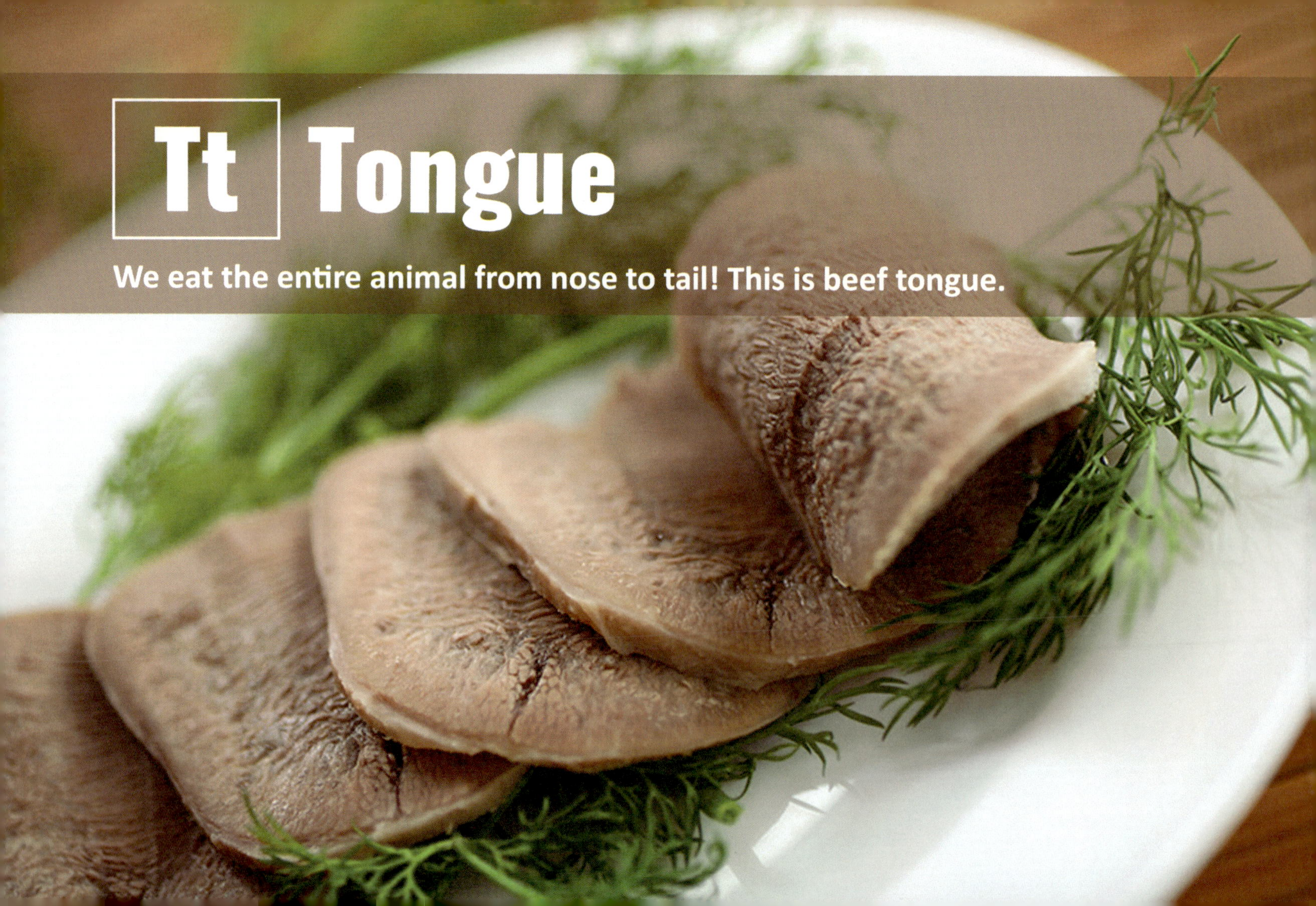

Tt Turkey

Turkey is traditionally eaten at Thanksgiving. We save the bones for broth!

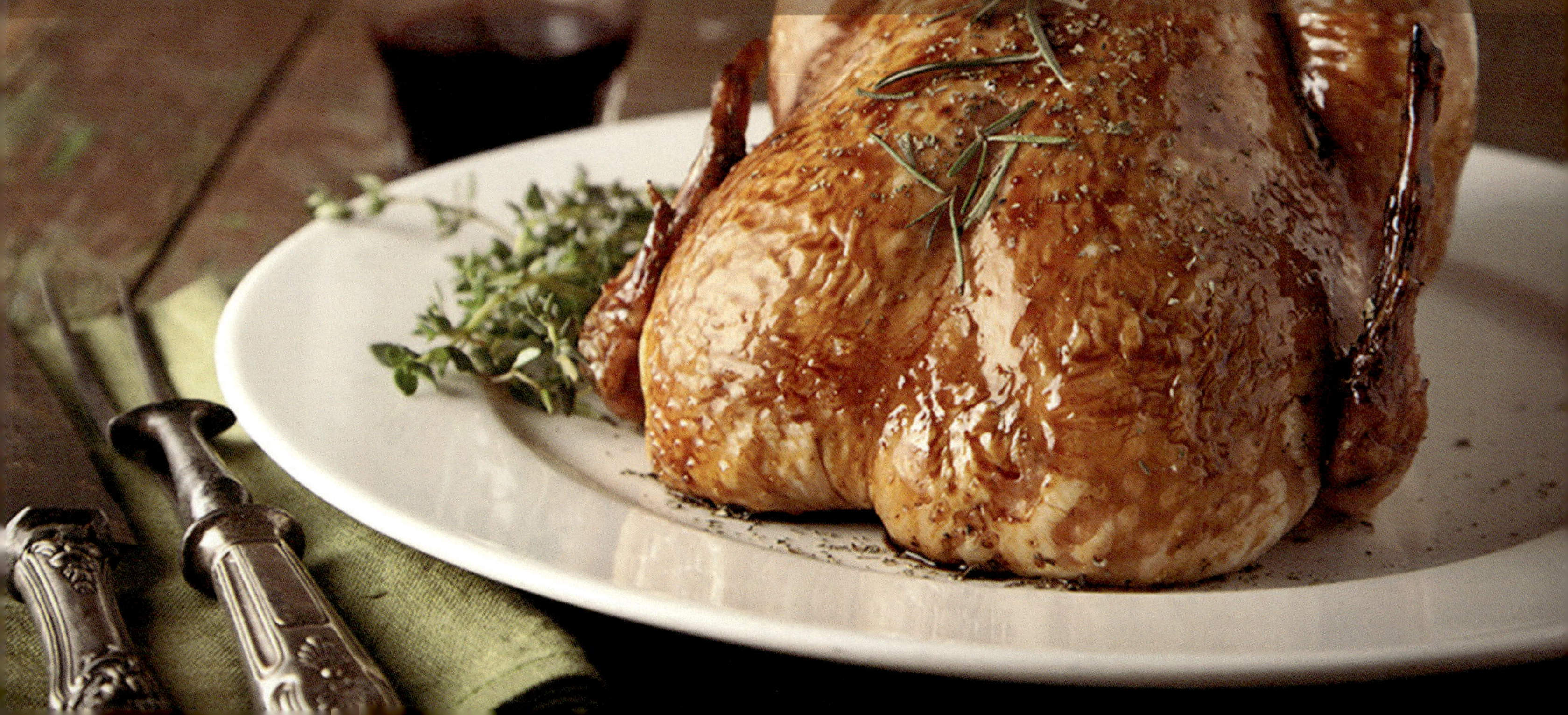

Un Unpasteurized Cheese

Cheese made from unheated milk is aged for at least 60 days.

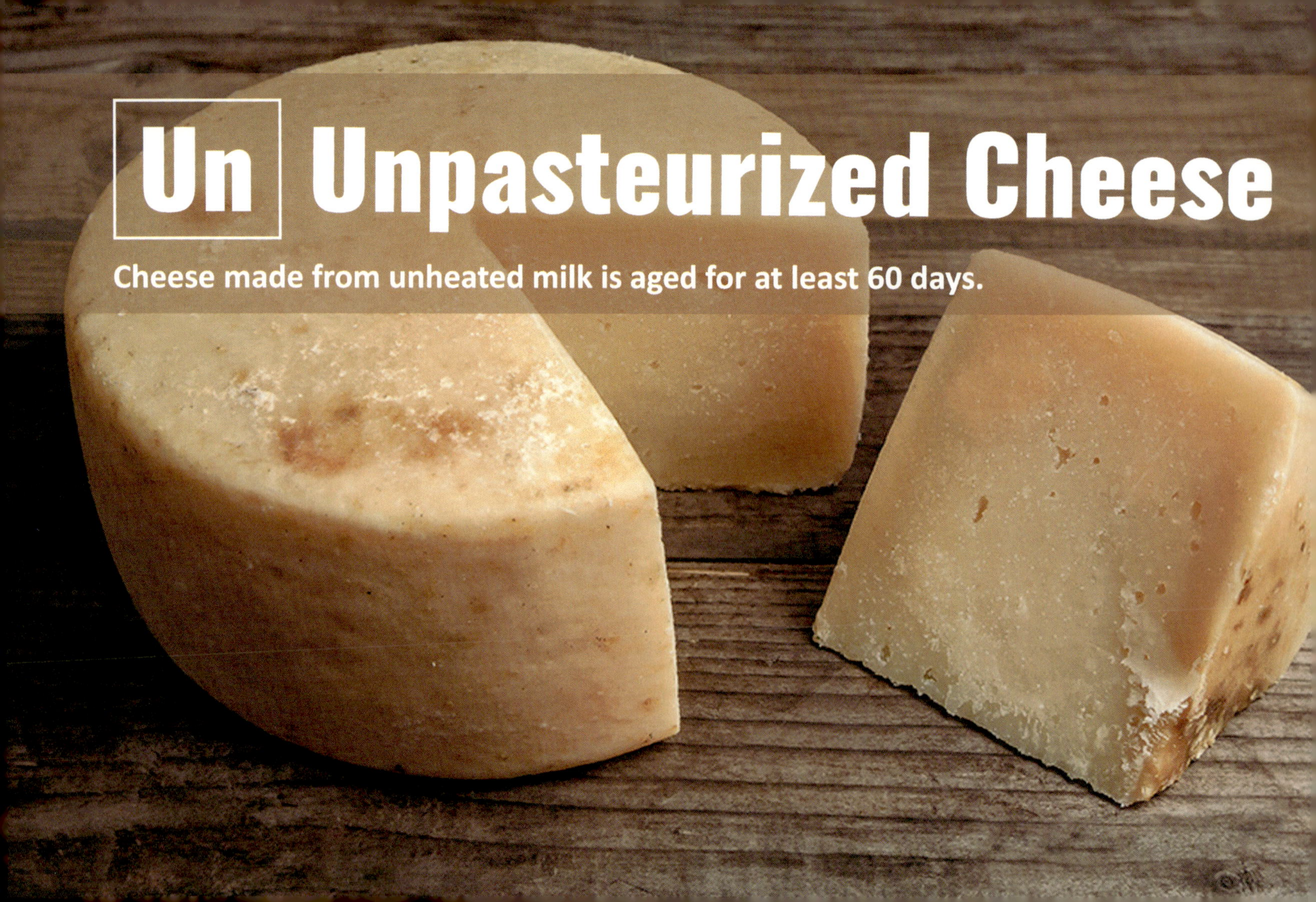

Un Unrefined Salt

Natural salt contains minerals needed by the body to function properly.

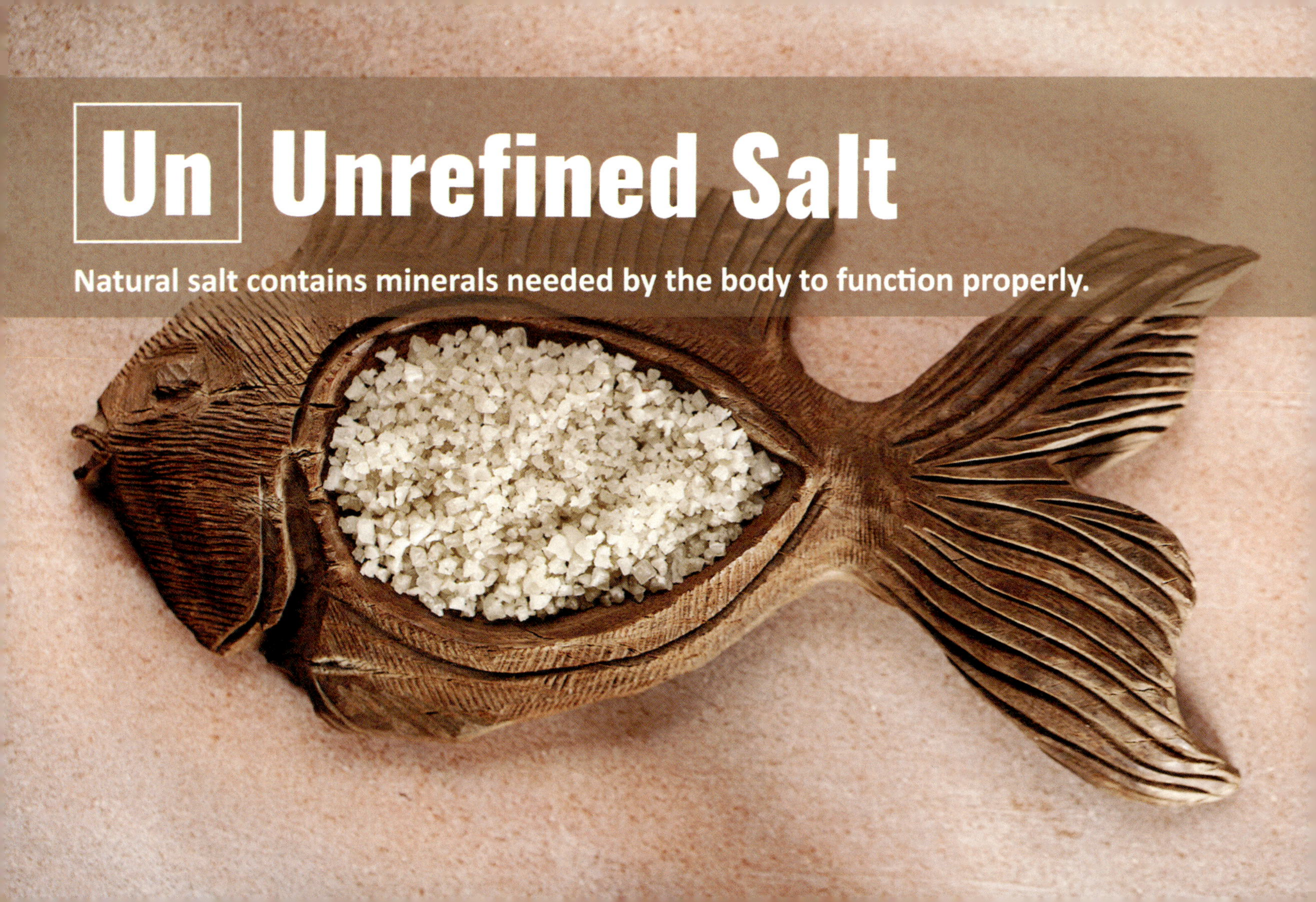

Vv Vanilla

Vanilla is a flavoring that comes from the fruit of an orchid plant called vanilla.

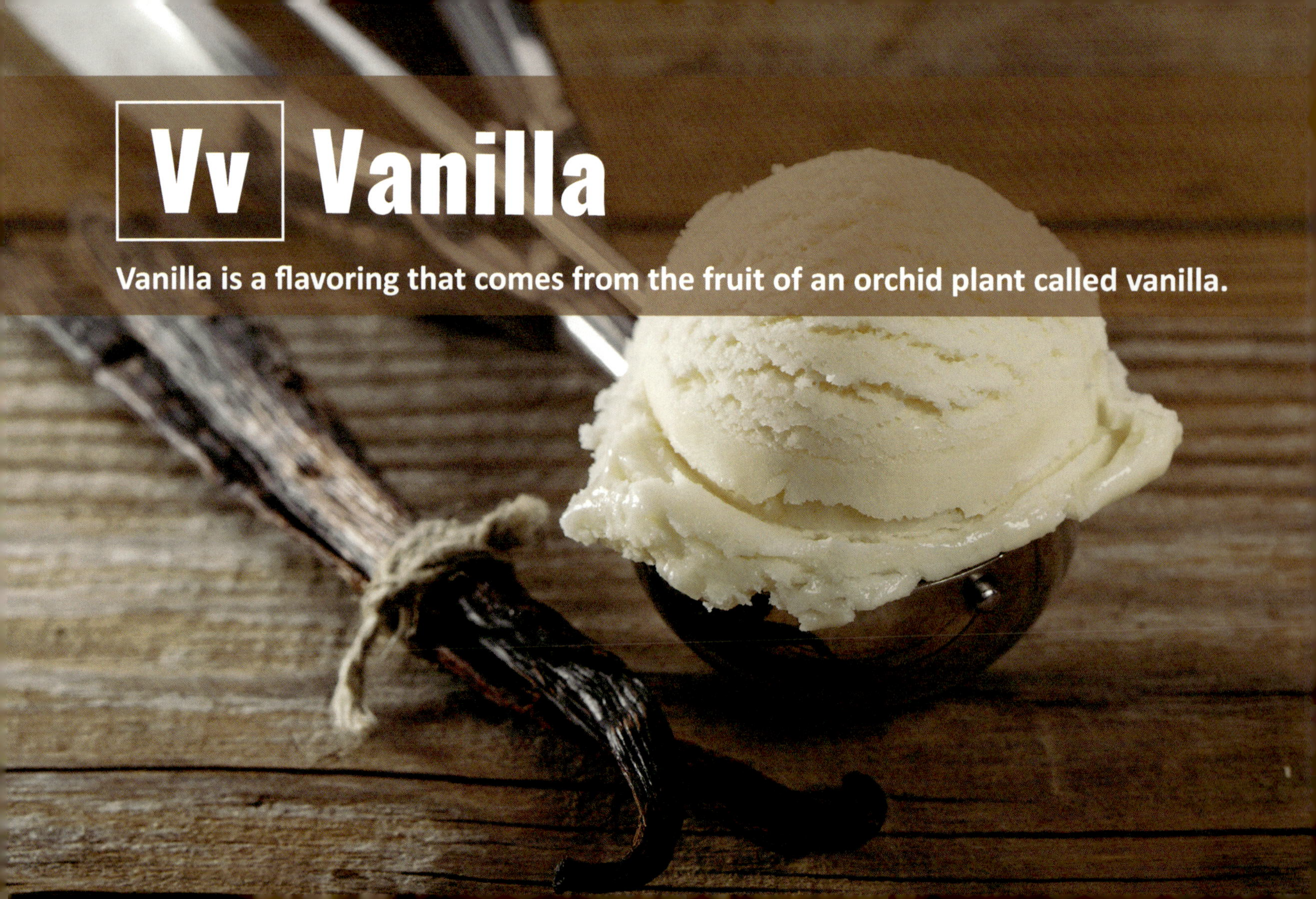

Vv Vinegar

There are different kinds of vinegar such as balsamic and apple cider vinegar.

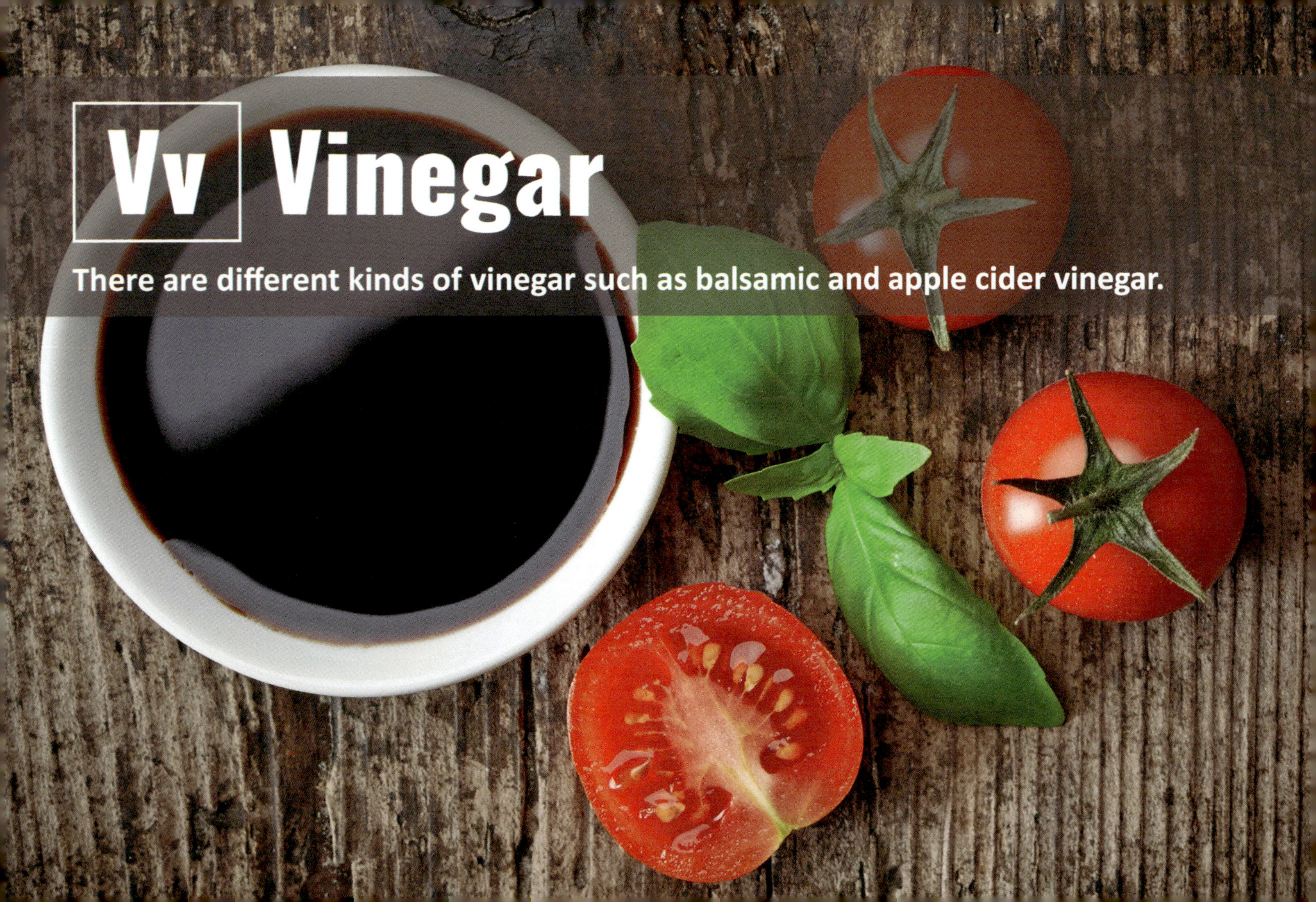

Ww Whey

Whey is the starter for lacto-fermented fruits, vegetables and beverages.

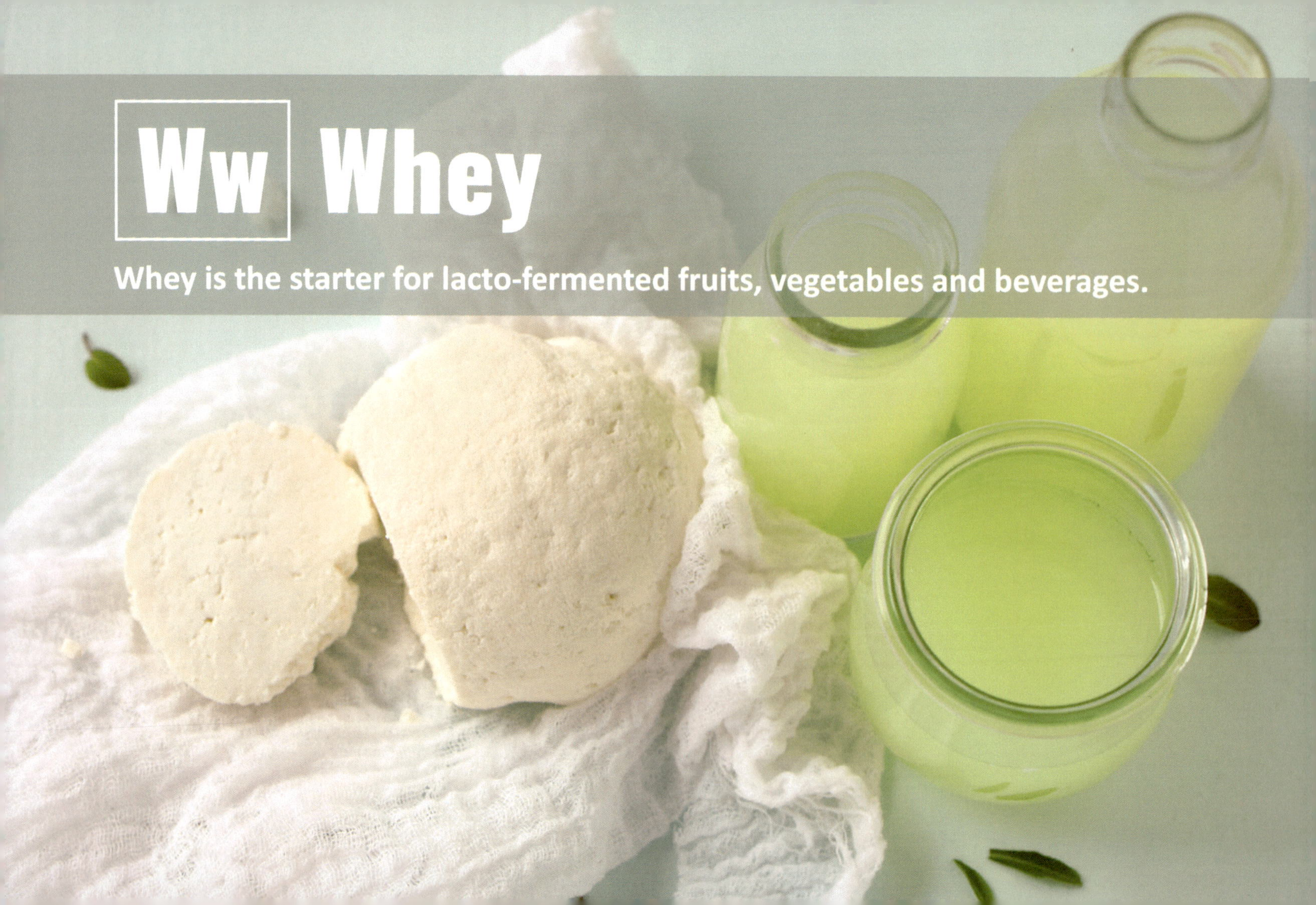

Ww Wild-Caught

Wild-caught fish and seafood are healthier for us to eat than farm-raised.

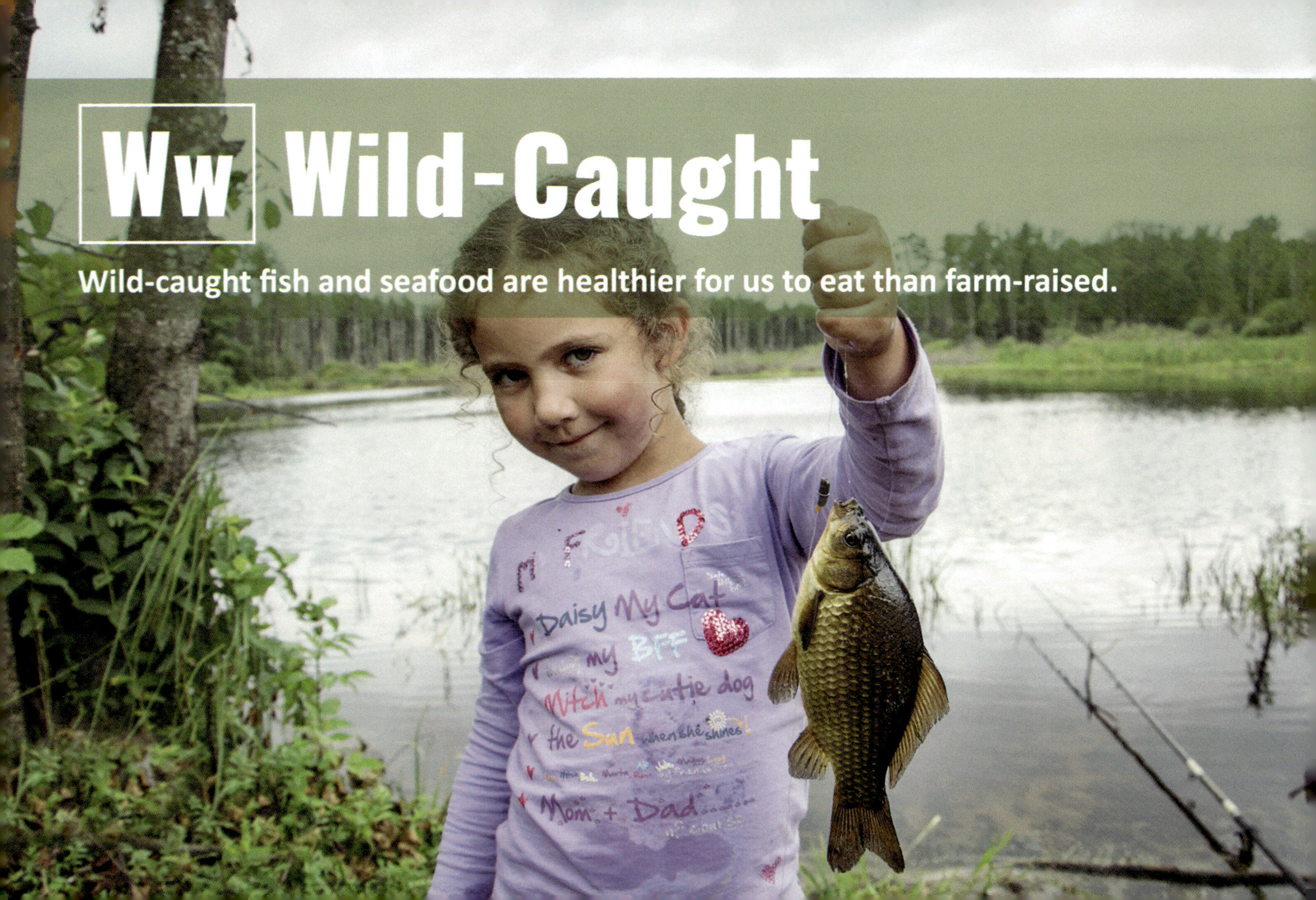

Xx Xigua

Xigua is the Chinese word for watermelon. Watermelon came from Africa.

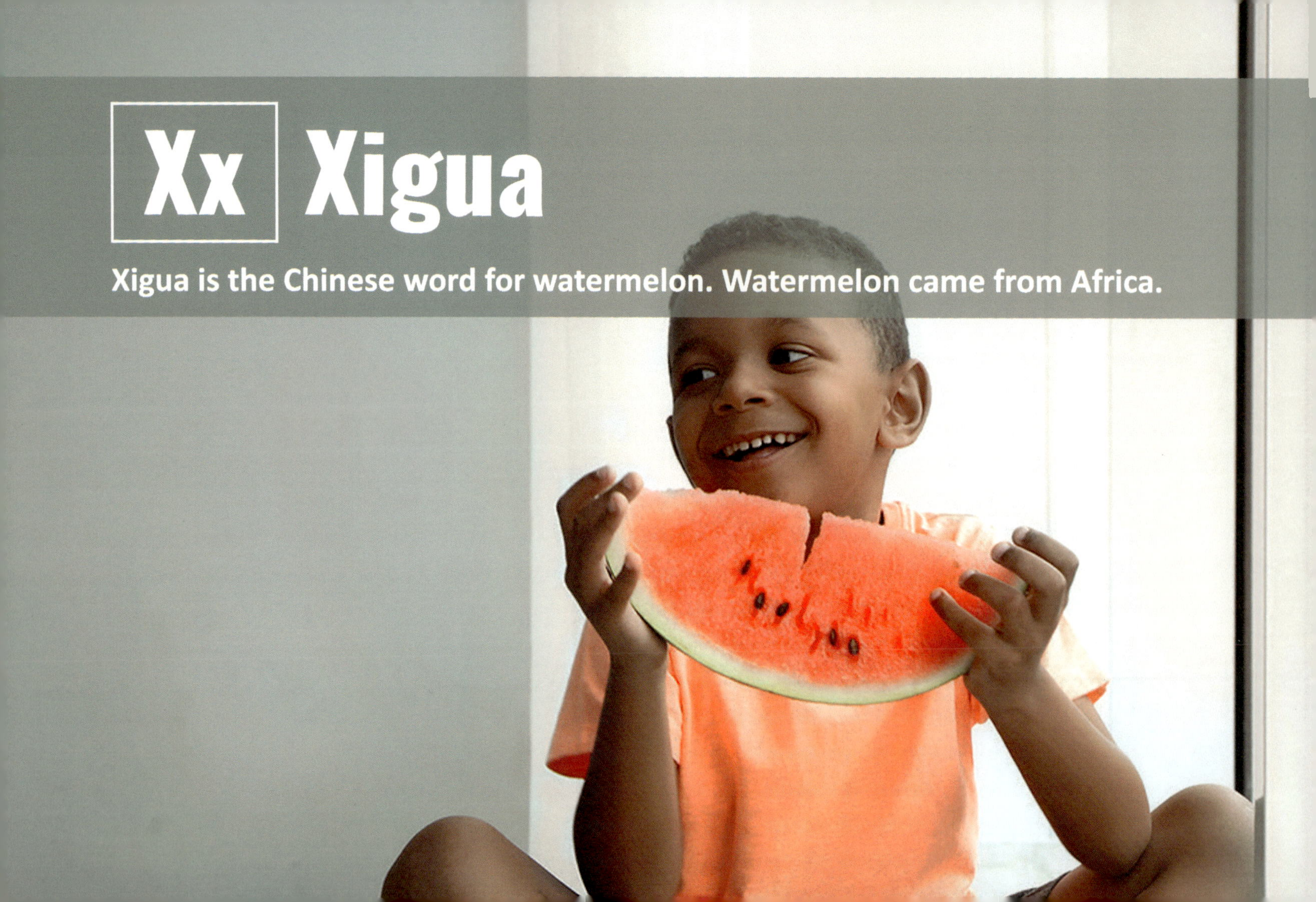

Xx Xoconostle

Xoconostle cactus fruit grows in central Mexico. Pronounced choko-nostlee.

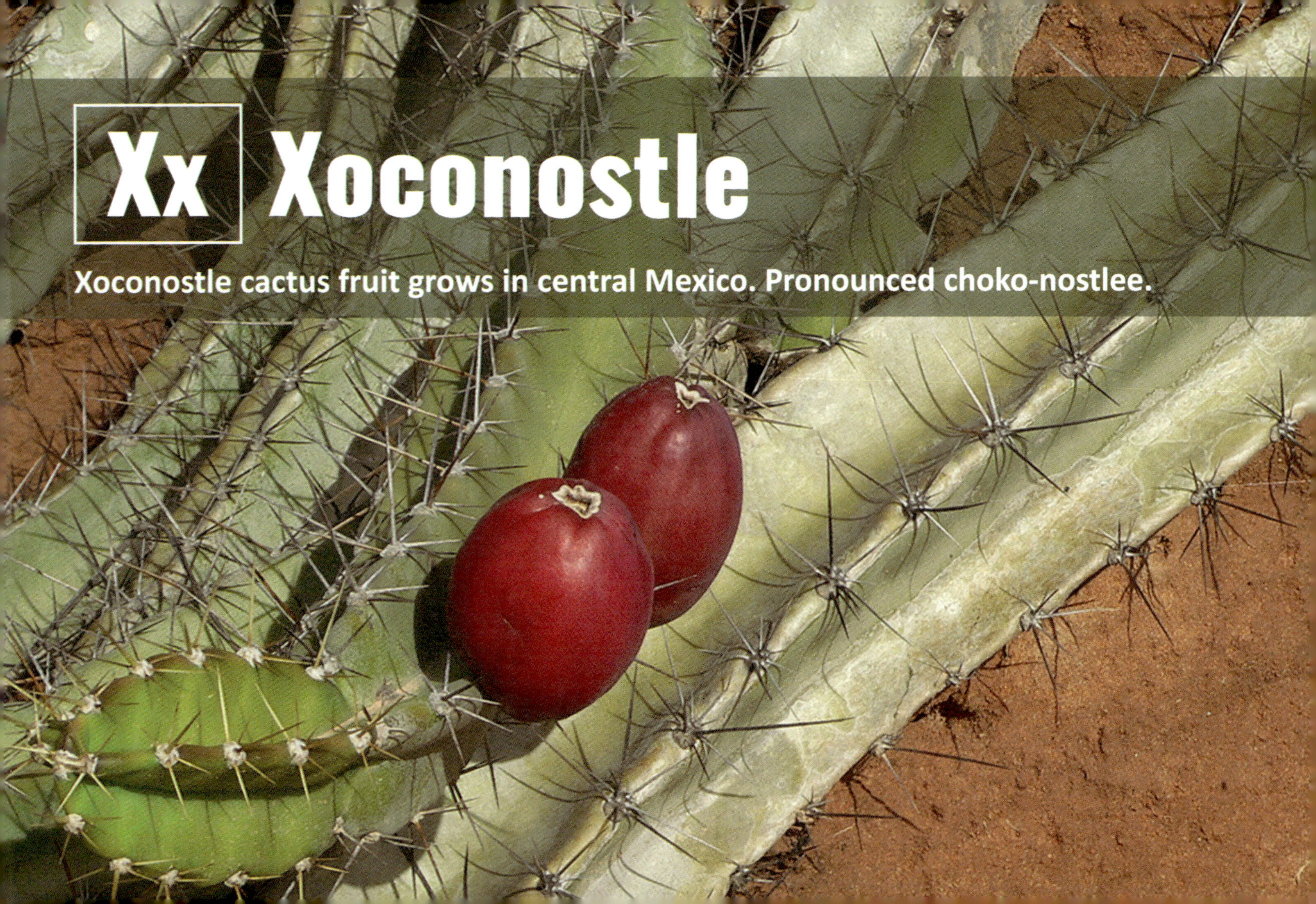

Yy Yams

While yams appear very similar to sweet potatoes, they're not even related.

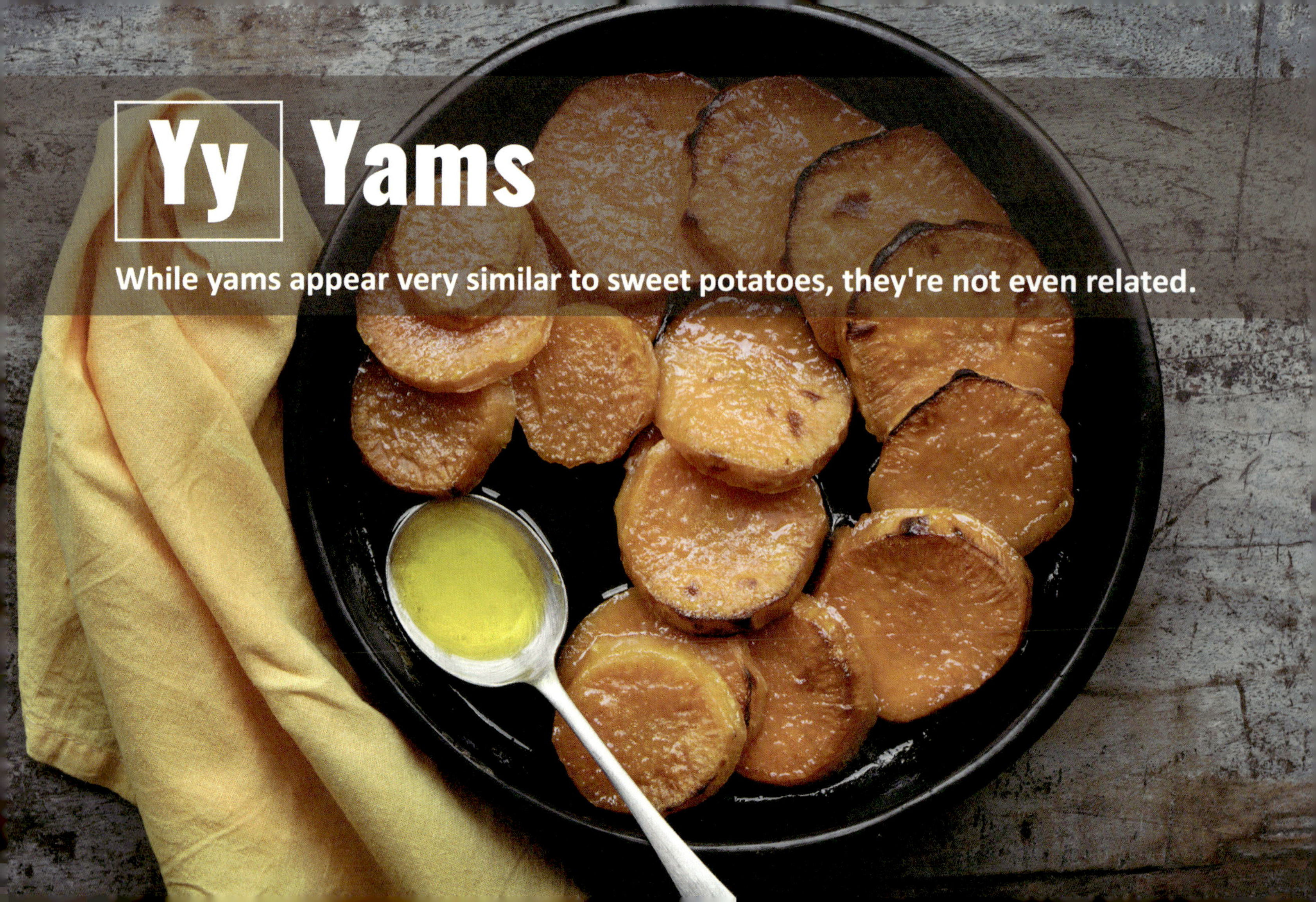

Yy Yogurt

Yogurt is cultured milk full of beneficial bacteria called probiotics.

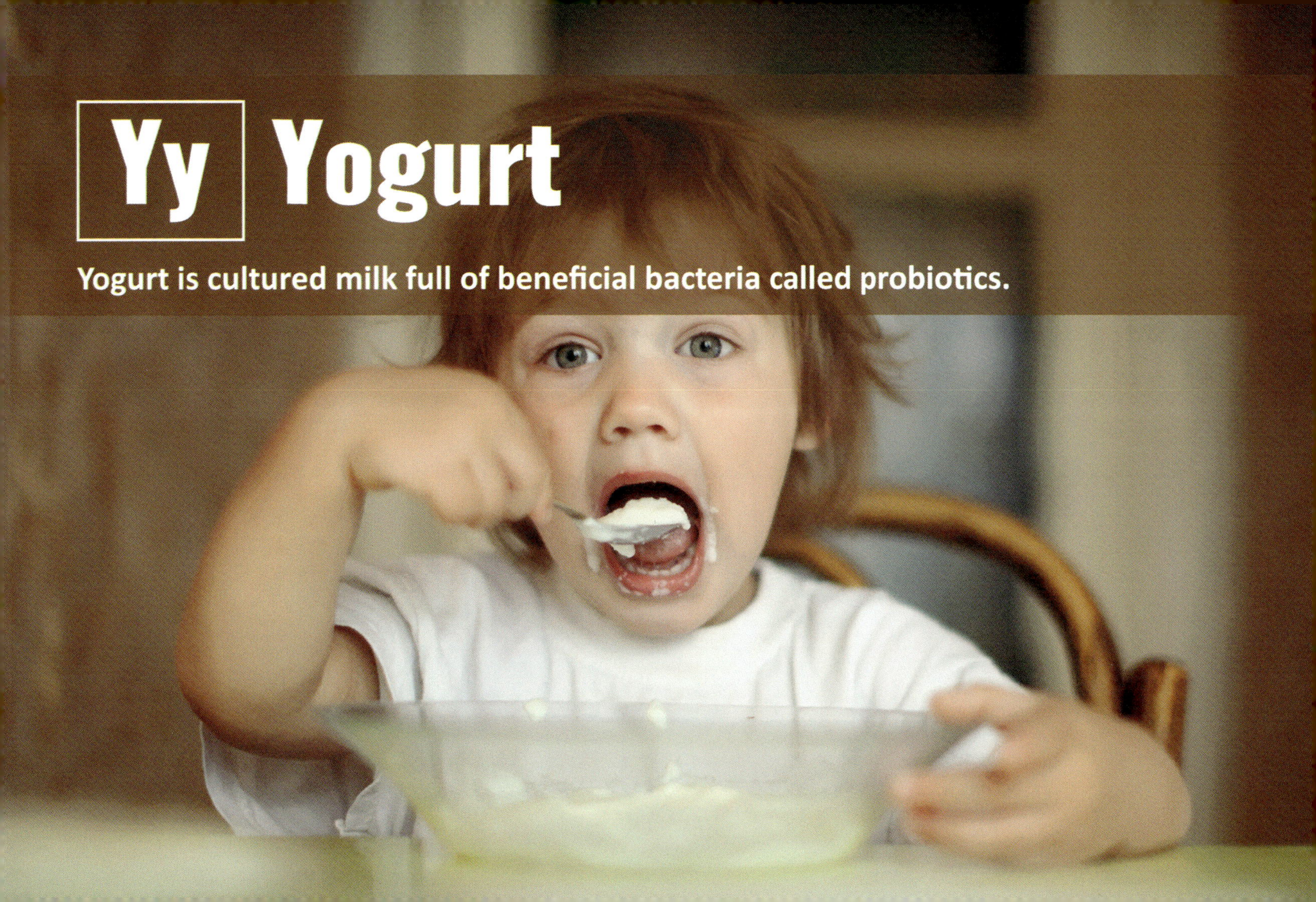

Zz Zest

Zest is the grated skin from oranges, limes and lemons added to dishes.

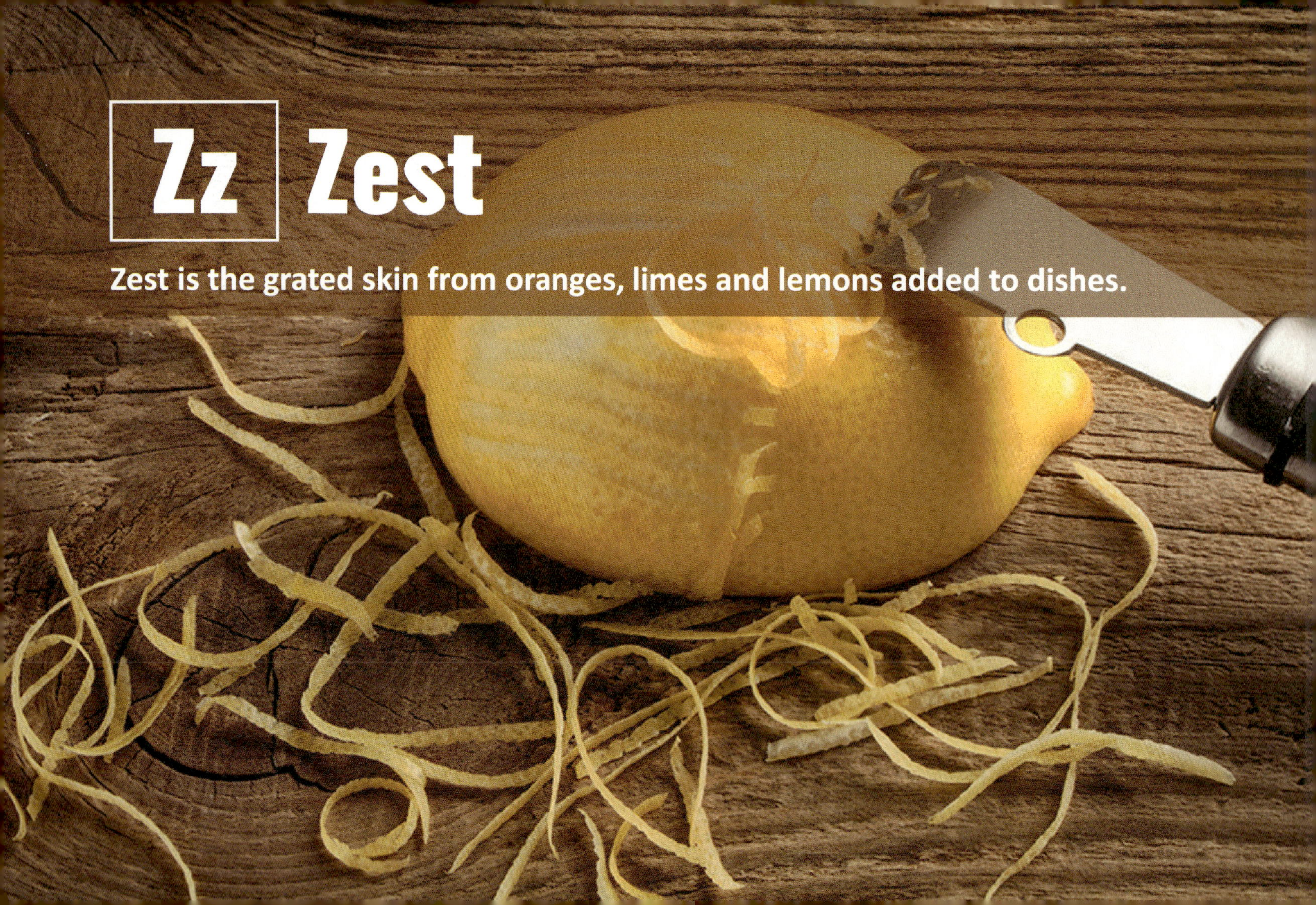

Zz Zucchini

Zucchini grows in warmer weather and comes in various shapes and colors.

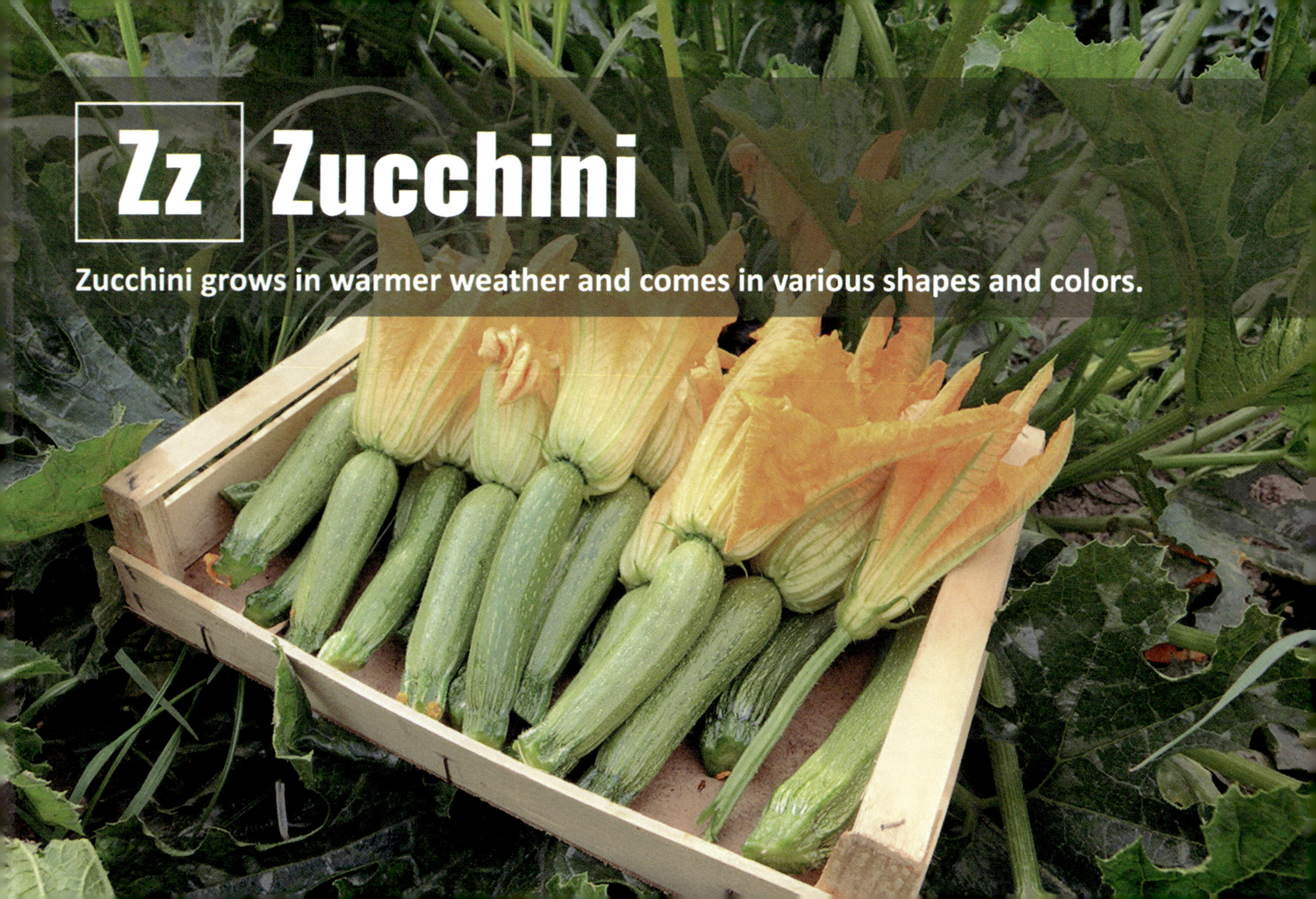

JOIN US

Learn more about the real food described in this book at nourishingourchildren.org/a-real-food-alphabet
Join us on Facebook at facebook.com/groups/arealfoodalphabet